S0-EAI-522

Health Care in the
People's Republic of China

About the Book and Author

The Chinese health care system is deeply rooted in a traditional, agricultural way of life, but since the late 1970s it has been increasingly influenced by the dynamics of a modernizing society. Dr. Rosenthal, using data collected through interviews, small-scale surveys, and the Chinese press, examines how Chinese medicine is being transformed. She describes how barefoot doctors are involved in a slow professionalization process, how traditional health care methods are being selectively integrated with western medicine, how the traditional pharmacopoeia is becoming patent medicine, and how recent market policy has introduced the practice of private medicine into the public system. Despite these advances, though, rural-urban disparities in the quality of health care are growing. Because modernization has emphasized the expansion of already advanced health facilities, rural health care, except for selected projects, is rapidly falling behind.

Marilynn M. Rosenthal is associate professor and medical sociologist in the Behavioral Sciences Department and director of the Program in Health and Society at the University of Michigan–Dearborn.

Health Care in the People's Republic of China

Moving Toward Modernization

Marilynn M. Rosenthal

Westview Press / Boulder and London

Westview Special Studies on China

Published in 1987 in the United States of America by Westview Press, Inc.; Frederick A. Praeger, Publisher; 5500 Central Avenue, Boulder, Colorado 80301

Library of Congress Cataloging-in-Publication Data
Rosenthal, Marilynn M.
Health care in the People's Republic of China.
   (Westview special studies on China)
   Includes index.
   1. Medical care—China.   2. Medicine, Chinese—China.
I. Title.   II. Series.   (DNLM: 1. Delivery of Health
Care—trends—China.   WA 395 R815h)
RA395.C53R67   1987   362.1′0951   86-32501
ISBN 0-8133-7365-4

Composition for this book was provided by the author.
This book was produced without formal editing by the publisher.

Printed and bound in the United States of America

The paper used in this publication meets the requirements of the American National Standard for Permanence of Paper for Printed Library Materials Z39.48-1984.

6   5   4   3   2

Dedicated to J.J., Addy, Al (1904–1986), Josh, Helen, Sue, Bob, Gary, Chris, Ellen, Richard, Harriet, Irv, Leslie, Marty, Andy, Pam, Elliot, Jackie, Jill, Sandy, Dan and Gregory—the family—filled with fun, warmth and caring

CONTENTS

TABLES AND FIGURES

TABLES

FIGURES

PREFACE

Striking changes are taking place in the health care system of the People's Republic of China, particularly in relation to its characteristics during and immediately after the Cultural Revolution.

This book captures the early phase of those changes, in the period of time shortly after the current modernization policies were announced and as they began to be implemented. The first five chapters of this book will provide the reader with the background necessary to understand what is taking place today. The sixth chapter, however, includes current material and brings the reader up-to-date.

Chapters One through Five are based primarily on material gathered in 1979 and 1981 during study courses on health care in the People's Republic of China. They describe and discuss the historical development of health policy and the health system, beginning with the Chinese Communist revolutionary success in 1949, and bring the reader to the early stages of the modernization process. In the late 1980s, the changes are accelerating; in the early 1980s, the health care system was just starting to respond and those early responses are reflected in the first five chapters of this book.

Hence, the book begins with a discussion of the slowly emerging efforts to professionalize the Barefoot Doctors and the new conceptualization of how they ought to change. Chapters Two and Five describe the extent to which the integration of Traditional and western medicine had actually taken place and the current push to standardize and transform Traditional herbs. Chapter Three explores the inequities in the rural health care delivery system, inequities further exacerbated by modernization policies today. The difficulties and challenges of the family planning program are discussed in Chapter Four. Not only is the program partially carried out in the health care sector, but its success is pivotal to the success of modernization in general.

These chapters of the book lead the reader through the foundations of the most recent changes to the final chapter, Chapter Six, which offers a summary overview of what is taking place today. In fact, the reader may want to begin with the last chapter and then return to the first five for a decade-long perspective that provides backdrop for current development.

One of the keys to the changes occurring throughout Chinese society as a whole is the Responsibility System which emphasizes individual and family enterprise and has stimulated the development of a private market sector. Collective and commune activities have subsided or even disappeared in many rural areas. This has had important implications for the health care system. These range from encouragement and creation of private medical practice to a disruption of the rural co-operative medical funds. It has also stimulated greater concern for quality of medical care and a desire for more and better medical technology as well as higher standards for existing practitioners and practices. Discussion of these can be found in Chapter Six.

China is a large and complex country and the modernization process will be a long and arduous one. It will take place neither evenly nor smoothly. Indeed, in many areas of the country, particularly poorer ones, the health care system will remain essentially as we saw it in 1979 and 1981. So while the most dramatic changes will continue to be noted and discussed, this book provides a picture of the diversity in the health care system. A diversity which will remain as the People's Republic of China moves slowly towards modernization.

Marilynn M. Rosenthal

ACKNOWLEDGMENTS

It was Peter M. New (1932–1986) who first encouraged me to analyze the voluminous material that had been gathered during my 1979 study course to the People's Republic of China. His interest, encouragement and enthusiasm sustained that effort for some period of time beginning with his invitation to organize a panel presentation of our material at the 1980 annual conference of the Society for Applied Anthropology. Peter also reviewed several of the articles in this book in their earlier drafts. His expertise was made available with considerable generosity, and his untimely death was a great loss to his family, friends, colleagues and the discipline to which he contributed.

A number of other people have been particularly helpful over the years these essays have been in the making. Charles Tilly helped me think through the first article that was written, "Political Process and the Integration of Traditional and Western Medicine." Marty Whyte seemed to direct me towards a new source of information at just the right moment on several occasions, and he also provided the hospitality of a desk at the Center for Research on Social Organizations at The University of Michigan where much of the writing for this book was undertaken. Sheila Hillier in London, in endless, extended and animated conversations over many summers, shared her tremendous knowledge of the Chinese health care system. David M. Lampton and Arthur Kleinman offered encouragement via letter that was most helpful. To all these colleagues, many, many thanks. I take full responsibility, however, for any perversions of their ideas and suggestions and, of course, for all the conclusions of this book.

A number of energetic students contributed immeasurably to this work. Paul Pongor and Jay Greiner, with whom I wrote two of the chapters, were the kind of students who make teaching a particular pleasure. They are now welcomed colleagues. Melissa Gregory, John Leung, Terri Turner, Jeff Soble, Rob Franchi and Wendy Yap provided invaluable help as research assistants and are also part of the health professional world now. All the students who enrolled in the 1979 and 1981 studies courses to the People's Republic of China were part of the effort to collect information. It was a delight to work with them in those special months preparing for and participating in the courses. The same must be said for students in my "Comparative Health Care Systems" course at The University of Michigan-Dearborn. Their enthusiasm and interest sustains my own.

Professor Charles Gliozzo, Director of Overseas Studies at Michigan State University, Vice Chancellor Eugene Arden of The University of Michigan-Dearborn and Kim Bruhn, who was Dean of UM-Dearborn's College of Arts, Science and Letters, all provided the institutional support needed to make the PRC study courses possible. I could not have done it without them. Catherine Arnott, Mary Dubuc, Nancy Lemkie, Mary Ann Rodgers and Donna Trupiano provided their usual high quality technical assistance.

A number of colleagues invited me to make presentations based on this material, and these talks helped me clarify my thinking in important ways. Edgar Borgenhammer at the Nordic School of Public Health in Gothenburg, Sweden, graciously let me take part in one of his outstanding conferences in 1983. Bill Kearns extended his special brand of exuberant hospitality for a presentation at the Department of Community Medicine, St. Marys Hospital Medical School in London. Richard Levinson, a much admired colleague at Emory University, arranged lectures there and at the Georgia Sociological Association. The Stockholm County Medical Services Board, endlessly generous to visiting scholars, listened patiently as I described the health care system in China. Finally, my colleagues and students at UM-D were the first to listen to our "Report to the Campus: Health Care in the PRC" presentation in the Fall of 1979. I thank you all for your kind invitations and consideration.

I hope it will be a special pleasure for all those who helped along the way to read the following pages and for others, as well, who might share our fascination with health care in the People's Republic of China.

M.M.R.

INTRODUCTION

As the People's Republic of China moves slowly towards modernization, how will its well-known health care system change?

A great deal has been written about the Chinese health care system, particularly in the late 1970s and early 1980s. Many articles and books described the unique features of the system: the use of peasants as Barefoot Doctors and the preservation and pervasive use of Chinese Traditional medicine as well as the mass campaigns to eliminate health problems. Many were intriqued by the slogan that personified health care policy after the revolution—Serve the People—bespeaking a determination to emphasize care to China's underserved masses especially in the rural countryside. While the first reports tended to romantize what was seen, scholars began to look more systematically and objectively at what was occurring in the health care system, although under limited research circumstances. Much of what has been described was a reflection of the Cultural Revolution and its aftermath. While more and more is appearing in scholarly journals about changes under the current modernization policies, little that is comprehensive has been brought together under one cover that focuses on the changes and particularly the change process. Perhaps this book will begin to fill that gap.

The modernization policies that now shape at least economic developments in the PRC have unfolded since the late 1970s and early 1980s. These policies include decollectivization of agricultural production emphasizing the "household system" of production contracts from the State, more autonomy in the management of various enterprises, particularly in industry, the far-reaching deregulation of prices, the stimulation of free enterprise in small industry, commerce and the service sector, and the opening of the country to more western contact. According to one of Europe's leading China scholars, Professor Jürgen Domes of Saar University, Germany,[1] these policies have produced some noteworthy results and some potential problems.

China's GNP has had an annual growth rate of 8.4 percent, grain production has increased 28 percent, the PRC has increased its share of world trade, village income has increased, in some rural areas more rapidly than urban incomes, and 20 percent of all peasant families have built new homes. The problems include a mounting foreign trade deficit, a depletion of China's foreign reserves and the development of increasing income differentials within rural villages.

What are the implications of these developments for the health care system?

Specifically, the stimulation of private enterprise has opened up the possibilities for private medicine, a startling development for anyone whose encounters with the Chinese health care system were in the 1970s. The shape of "privatization" remains to be described although it has been reported that in 1986, 116,000 doctors, dentists and nurses were involved in the delivery of private medical care (3.5 percent of health personnel). Of greater importance in the modernization process is the opening up of more western contact and growing acceptance of western models. An element of this is the larger meaning of modernization itself with its emphasis on advanced technology, science, technical expertise and both specialization and standardization.

All of these manifestations of modernization will have their impact on the upgrading and professionalization of medical personnel including the famous Barefoot Doctors, on the westernization (in various forms) of Chinese Traditional medicine, on the push for standardization of pharmaceutical products, and improved quality of care. Furthermore, as the pace of modernization is different around the country, the ability to achieve equity in health care delivery will be effected. Inequities already in the system will be exacerbated particularly in rural areas of the country. The ability to implement the family planning program, particularly in the more Traditional rural countryside, becomes a key factor in the modernization process. All of these are explored in this book.

Chinese health policy evolves within the same general framework that shapes every national health policy: political ideology and economic resources. As these have changed, health policy has changed but always with roots in previous historical developments. Health policy is usually one of the instruments of the larger, dominating political ideology and China has been no exception. Chinese health policy has also been the product of the interplay between various interest groups as in other nations. This has been eloquently described in David Lampton's *The Politics of Chinese Medicine* which informs several of the essays in this collection. And it shall be seen that China has struggled to deal, often in unique ways, with the same problems facing all health care systems. Equity, access, uniform financing, distribution of resources, quality of care.

Modernization is a long and a slow process. It has been predicted that if China's growth rate continues as it has in the last few years, for the next thirty years, it will have achieved the level of development of Poland. As for the health care system, it will remain for a long time to come, a continuum of the simple clinics and health campaigns of the years of the Socialist Transformation and Great Leap Forward, the Barefoot Doctors and impetus for Traditional medicine of the Cultural Revolution, and the westernization brought with current modernization efforts. For a long time to come it will be constrained by lack of resources and the inability to provide equity of access to the same standards of care all over the country.

It will, at the same time, continue to command the interest and attention of those interested in comparative health care policy and comparative health care systems. Not so that specific programs or unique approaches can be imitated; these are too culture-bound and historically circumscribed. But rather to capture a new picture of the modernization process itself.

Rather than presenting information in an ideological context, this book is a more systematic, sociological description and discussion. It provides a relatively objective "snapshot" of

4

a health care system rooted in traditional agricultural society but increasingly influenced by the dynamics of modern society. The result is a unique Chinese version of the modernization process.

There are lessons to be learned from an understanding of health care policy and implementation in the People's Republic of China. They are the subtle lessons of how to innovate within the context of one's own culture and resources. They are the lessons of using political power and determination. And they are the lessons of using the larger social structure to deal with health problems.

The material in this book was gathered from a variety of sources. These include information gathering during two health care study courses to the People's Republic of China in 1979 and 1981 that permitted short interviews, small scale surveys and systematic observations based on comprehensive and intensive reviews of the literature before leaving for China. Information obtained in the PRC was dependent on translations provided by the guides and translators who accompanied the groups. The groups however, did include individuals who spoke and understood Chinese. The complete journals of both the 1979 and 1981 study groups contain transcriptions of all information gathered and are available upon request. Appendix A lists all places visited in 1979 and 1981. Original material gathered in this fashion has been used in conjunction with extensive literature reviews that have included scholarly journals and books, American newspapers like *The New York Times* and *Wall Street Journal* as well as summaries of *Mainland China Press* through 1986.

NOTE
1. Domes, Jürgen, "The Politics of Economic Reforms in the PRC: Politics, Results and Future Perspectives." Presentation at the Center for Chinese Studies, The University of Michigan, Ann Arbor, Michigan, 9 March 1987.

1
THE BAREFOOT DOCTORS OF CHINA: FROM POLITICAL CREATION TO PROFESSIONALIZATION

with Jay Greiner

China's Barefoot Doctor program is undergoing significant change. Since 1977, the numbers have declined from 1,760,000 to 1,575,000, with 185,000 dismissed as incompetent or leaving for other reasons. Standards for training are rising with increased emphasis on medical work; a two-level system of examinations has been instituted. This includes a BFD competency test and a more advanced examination to receive certification as a "country or village doctor" for the best students. A small percentage of medical school places is to be reserved for the most promising. Overall, current policy indicates BFDs are to become the equivalent of three-year medical school graduates (assistant doctors), be full-time practitioners and receive salaries instead of workpoints (Chen 1981:29–31; Taylor 1980:23; Mainland China Press 1981).

These recent changes in China's Barefoot Doctor policy suggest a need for reappraisal of the program as a medical manpower strategy. This article will briefly review the historical roots of the BFD program, summarize the research literature, add new material collected during 1979 and 1981 study courses in the PRC and offer a current assessment of this unique policy.

It is now well known that in June of 1965, on the eve of the Great Proletariate Cultural Revolution, Chairman Mao announced a new health policy: a Barefoot Doctor program designed to deal with the continuing shortage of physicians for China's vast rural population. Mao mandated that hundreds of thousands of rural peasants, chosen by their work comrades, would be given several months of rudimentary medical training. They would continue in agricultural labor part-time in addition to serving the elementary health care needs of their fellow workers.

Original BFD Policy

This was a remarkable idea in its daring and in its risks. Based on early efforts during the 1930s Rural Reconstruction Movement (Lucas 1980:461–89) and small 1950s experiments near Shanghai (Rifkin 1973:147), the Barefoot Doctor policy appeared to have a number of purposes: (1) It created a new health provider category to deal with both the continuing shortage and maldistribution of physicians. Despite successful efforts both to increase the number of medical students and to disperse them to rural areas, the stark doctor shortage so evident in 1949 at the point of liberation continued, as did the urban clustering of the medical profession. (2) Mao's anger with the medical profession, one of the urban elites he had always mistrusted, had reached new heights. He attacked the Ministry of Health with intense fury in 1965. It was one of the power bases of his political enemies and represented resistance to his conception of the principles of continuing revolution. By creating a large cadre of health workers from outside the world of professional medical knowledge, he moved to undercut professional control of medical work.

Three, Mao and the Chinese Communist Party (CCP) still had unfulfilled and important obligations to the rural masses who had made the revolution a success. The Barefoot Doctor concept was a bold move to make good on promises in a dramatic, egalitarian manner: taking young peasants, training them, yet leaving them to continue working alongside of their comrades in the fields. This ingenious idea would cause a minimum drain on agricultural workers where all hands are needed. It also fortified the concept of equal status between the practitioner and the patient. (4) Further, the policy emphasized local autonomy and initiatives, consistent with the 1960s thrust for decentralization. (5) Finally, it was a concrete example of the Cultural Revolution's emphasis on practical work rather than theoretical education.

This new medical manpower policy also reflected a continuation of Mao's original principles of health work: Barefoot Doctors were to be trained in both western and Traditional medical knowledge, to practice preventive medicine, to organize their fellows in mass health campaigns and serve the health needs of people at the grass roots level. In essence, it was a reiteration, in 1965, of the four principles enunciated in 1950. It was an idea of political and revolutionary significance, but certainly not appealing to professional medicine and professional biomedical education standards.

Contention between Mao's and the CCP's concept of health work, and the ideas of the medical profession with its power base in the Ministry of Health, had a history that began in 1949 and continued until Mao's death in 1976. The ongoing battle over health policy and its actual implementation was between a revolutionary, political apparatus anxious to harness ideological fervor to solve problems quickly and a bureaucratized profession given to slow, rational behavior, scientific standards and validation, and a very large measure of autonomy in its work. Lampton (1977:250–273) has written in detail about the political struggles between the two approaches.

The Ministry of Health was willing and able to increase enrollments in medical schools, shorten medical education to a certain extent, and increase the physician manpower supply in this manner. But it wanted to do so in a way that maintained certain standards for medical education and medical practice. And like physicians everywhere, they preferred to practice in urban centers where technology, research, and peer support were available, even if minimal. Such an approach was not capable of producing the numbers of doctors needed for the vast Chinese rural countryside.

Mao and the CCP, on the other hand, needed to enhance the rural collectivization efforts, strengthen the burgeoning rural cooperative medical services, and stem the flood of rural peasants to the already overburdened urban medical facilities. Mao's BFD policy took the issue of increased and better distributed medical manpower out of the professional arena and into the political.

The overall medical manpower pool in the PRC encompasses seven categories of health workers (Cheng 1973:139–157). These include western-style doctors, assistant doctors, medical assistants, technical assistants, Traditional doctors, Barefoot Doctors, and health aides. Medical manpower figures at these various levels and at various time periods have been approximated and are included in Table 1.1. (See chapter appendix for this and all tables in this book). It is within the context of this array of medical personnel that Barefoot Doctors have been developed.

Literature Review

Descriptions of Barefoot Doctors have appeared in scholarly reports and journals (Sidel and Sidel 1973:78–88; Hsu 1974:113–127; New 1974:220–224) and the popular press since 1972. These reports inspired great interest and enthusiasm and were used by some to promote the idea of medical paraprofessionals to deal with the shortage of general practitioners and the general maldistribution of physicians in the American health care system. These initial reactions were often based on a superficial understanding of both the policy and its differential implementation.

The original BFD model recruits were chosen by local brigades and the people whom they would serve. Political awareness, interest in health, willingness to work conscientiously, and experience as an auxiliary health worker were usually prime qualifications; educational level was not considered of great importance although Barefoot Doctor candidates were generally middle-school graduates. The nature and length of training programs were highly variable in contrast to training programs for other levels of medical workers. Typically, there was a short-term course for three months to one year offered by the commune health center doctors that provided a brief introduction to medical knowledge. Special texts were usually prepared, perhaps by a provincial medical college. County health bureaus might also contribute educational material on local disease patterns. In-service training on a rotation basis provided additional medical education. Ideally, there was continuing education on a regular basis to build on the initial period of education. The initial policy regarding training officially called for a great deal of flexibility in the training programs to make them responsive to local interest, local economics, and local needs.

Unlike other levels of medical workers, Barefoot Doctors have not received wages but have been paid in workpoints like the agricultural workers who are their peers and their patients. Usually their workpoints are calculated by taking the average of the highest points for the brigade. Presumably, they were to do manual labor one-third to one-half of their time.

Medical work responsibility fell into several categories: overseeing environmental sanitation, rehabilitative care for discharged patients, immunization programs of various sorts, and the treatment of minor or common illnesses like colds, fever, eye infections, digestive tract and upper respiratory tract diseases, influenza, parasitic disease, and minute sprains and injuries. The immunization programs include systematic immunization for preschoolers and sporadic seasonal programs for the entire population. Because of their closeness to their patients, they were able to be available at work and for home and night visits. Environmental sanitation work included the control of water and waste, animal pens, and seasonal patriotic health campaigns. They also supervised aides who assisted them in this work as well as in first-aid administration.

As many observers have noted, this health care worker, unique to China, reflected an unusual medical concept combining some of the functions of doctor, nurse, and sanitation engineer but at a close, grass roots level, as a "neighborhood" medical worker. This, of course, describes the "ideal" or normative policy. The "reality" or action policy turns out to be something else. One of the most comprehensive and systematic studies of action policy is Tsui's research on health care delivery at two rural communes in Guangdong Province, which included observations of the role of the Barefoot Doctors and ascertained the extent to which they approximated the ideal model (Tsui 1979:129–156). She found some significant variations, which correlated with the economic level of a particular commune and its proximity to an urban center. Tsui's findings indicate that poorer, more remote communes are less able to support the Barefoot Doctor program. For example, they offer shorter initial training programs, and fewer and more variable in-service training for fewer Barefoot Doctors. Other observers (Lampton 1978:526–539; New 1975:239; Wang 1975:476–486) have written extensively on disparities in the rural health care system as well, noting that more remote areas are less well served and the ability of a commune and its production brigades to support Barefoot Doctors and the cooperative medical services is closely tied to agricultural output in any single year. The quality of BFDs is therefore relative to the ability to (1) spare agricultural workers, even part-time; (2) allocate sufficient resources and time to education and training; and (3) sustain an adequate level of continuing training.

Wang (1975:476–486) was able to systematize material she collected on the education and skill of BFDs in a number of communes, and she suggests that three models of training and practice exist. The three models represent a progressive movement on a continuum from preventive to curative care, and might be seen as signifying different stages of rural health service development.

THREE BFD TRAINING MODELS; STAGES IN RURAL HEALTH CARE

Model One. This model represents the minimum level of training and expertise a BFD has within the PRC health care system. The BFDs at this level are peripheral workers with very limited medical responsibilities, in part because of close proximity to other more advanced health facilities. A significant portion of their time is spent on environmental and sanitation work. The length of training ranges from one to three months. Much of the training is work practicum under supervision of a physician. Primary responsibilities are giving vaccinations, treating common illnesses, health education through the patriotic health campaigns, and family planning. Contraceptive pills are dispensed to women after an examination by the Barefoot Doctor. Referrals are frequently made to adjacent commune hospitals.

Model Two. This stage represents a moderate level of training and expertise. These Barefoot Doctors are more directly involved in patient care at the commune hospital level. This functions as a transitional health delivery approach at the commune hospital until fully trained physicians or a team of rotating physicians can be acquired. The length of training basically appears to be the same as in Model One, however, more practicum training under supervision of a physician occurs, especially in more medically advanced areas of surgery and internal medicine. Primary reponsibilities are the same as in Model One, except some of the BFDs at the commune hospital are especially trained to perform surgery such as appendectomies, repair of hernias, and vasectomies.

Model Three. This stage represents more development at a lower level in the rural services system. At this level there are physicians and secondary-level graduate physicians (assistant doctors) at the commune hospital, with the Barefoot Doctors being the practitioners at the production brigade level. The length of training at this stage is a minimum of six months. This training is more formal and occurs at the district hospital. Following this initial training, the hospital conducts in-service training one-half to one full day per week depending on the time or season of the year. Primary responsibilities include treatment of common illnesses, using surgery, internal medicine, dermatology, first aid, and emergency medical care. After two years of accrued training, the Barefoot Doctor can perform more complex medical procedures and treatment. The total training then, is two and one-half to three years in length. Barefoot Doctors at this stage are also involved in the training of health aides who receive two to three months of training, primarily in first aid and sanitation work.

Kleinman and Mechanic (1979:22–24) corroborate these three models functioning at the three tiers of delivery. However, they note an important problem of utilization, observing that numbers of patients bypass BFDs at the team and brigade level and seek care by better-trained personnel at higher levels. They suggest that this pattern reflects lack of confidence in the skills of Models One and Two BFDs. The authors also express concern about BFD medical judgement, based on observed diagnostic work of questionable thorough-ness, and drugs (e.g., chloramphenical) available to the Barefoot Doctors but not necessarily suited to their technical judgement. Kleinman comments that the large numbers of hospital in-patients they saw with rheumatic heart disease and nephritis may indicate not enough attention to streptoccocal infections at the primary level for which Barefoot Doctors have responsibility.

Other reports have raised questions about the quality of BFD care as well (Lampton 1977:237; Hsu 1974:124–127), linking the ability of the BFD to the level of agricultural prosperity and stability. Overall then, observations establish wide variations in the implementation of the BFD program that include (1) length of training, (2) time spent in medical work, (3) level of services delivered, and (4) quality of care. Further, there appears to be an inverse relationship between qualifications and services rendered. Finally, there are hints that patients skip the BFD tiers and continue to overutilize higher levels of care.

These astute observations have clearly been recognized in the PRC. The latest BFD policy changes appear to address precisely the issues raised in the reports summarized above.

Updating the Literature

The following information, based on observations and interviews conducted in 1979 and 1981, provides an opportunity to assess the gradual development and implementation of the most recent BFD policy statements. It is based on a policy briefing at the China Medical Association (Beijing Branch 1979), visits to three suburban communes, two "distant rural" communes, several county hospitals, as well as an urban, advanced-care hospital.

The Barefoot Doctor Situation in 1979

Our first day in Beijing on 12 August began with a general health care policy briefing at the China Medical Association (Study Journal 1979:23–40). Our hosts emphasized the continued and prime importance of the Barefoot Doctors in delivering health care in the countryside. Mention was also made of the continued need for the Barefoot Doctor to make an agricultural contribution to his or her work unit. The statement was phrased in an interesting manner: "The Barefoot Doctors," said the speaker, "are not adverse to productive labor so they [will continue as] part-time medical workers because of the economic conditions in the rural areas. If they are full-time, if they are divorced from productive labor, the peasants cannot show their responsibility economically. However, if their communes are wealthy enough, they can be released for full time medical work."

While reiterating this, the CMA spokesman went on to state that current policy calls for upgrading the "technological skills" of the worker doctors, by 1985, to the level of those trained in secondary medical schools.[2] This additional training, we were told, will be the responsibility of local county hospitals. The Barefoot Doctor training will continue to be a combination of Traditional and western techniques, but with a heavy reliance on Traditional herbs and acupuncture. However, the main duties of the Barefoot Doctors remain in prevention, particularly the "two controls and five improvements." This refers to the "control" of drinking water and night soil and the "improvement" of wells, animal pens, stoves, latrines, and the environment.

Part of our discussion focused on whether upgrading the education of these health workers would change their function. Would they soon be qualified to do other more complex and more sophisticated work? The response was ". . . the technical skills will be greatly increased, but their tasks are still the same." When asked whether this might stimulate dissatisfaction among Barefoot Doctors, that they would be overtrained for their level of job expectation, the response was that the better Barefoot Doctors could go on to the medical schools and the universities. We were told there has been a recent revival of national exams for medical university admission and that those Barefoot Doctors who had a middle-school education would be most able to compete on these examinations.[3]

Discussion of CMA briefing. A close look at the China Medical Association statement of the evolving policy regarding Barefoot Doctors suggests an inherent contradiction. The current program of increased technical education for Barefoot Doctors and the systematic upgrading of their technical skills (to Model Three) is consistent with the new emphasis on modernization and the new interest in broadening educational opportunity throughout the society. It is also an attempt to address the criticism of Barefoot Doctor qualifications. The fact that Barefoot Doctors should also continue to perform their same level of work suggests that training programs, to date, may have left a great deal to be desired and that criticism about quality of care is justified. This should not be considered surprising since the task of providing technical training to tens of thousands of poorly educated peasants is a formidable endeavor.

The inherent contradiction is that at the same time the training will become elaborated, Barefoot Doctors will continue to be asked to do agricultural work. While contributing to the agricultural economy, this distracts from the development of technical skills. Such division of time, energy, and attention works against the professionalization process that the new policy dictates. Perhaps an interesting bellweather of growth in agricultural productivity will be the extent to which Barefoot Doctors become full-time practitioners. It will also be important to see whether Barefoot Doctors will have a new career ladder to follow. The new educational program should open the way for more of them to qualify for advanced training and make the Barefoot Doctors more competitive on the national exams. The new educational program of secondary-level medical training also puts them into more contact with physicians of advanced training and hence emphasizes models for emulation and continuing socialization to physician norms. Suggested, therefore, is a strengthening of control over Barefoot Doctors by the medical profession.

Implied in the CMA briefing is the likelihood that BFDs as a group will become more stratified with many remaining at Model One levels (albeit with improved training), while those more proficient at the medical components of their work move up to the assistant doctor level and significantly increase the medical manpower pool in that category. It is hard to see how these latter Barefoot Doctors can also continue to do agricultural labor.

This briefing provided illuminating background as we met BFDs in various communes and as we gathered information about BFD education programs.

5th May Commune: Suburban BFD (Model Three). Our visit to the 5/3 (Third of May) Commune in suburban Shenyang included a visit to the commune hospital and an opportunity to speak with one of the commune's ninety Barefoot Doctors (Study Journal 1979:87–96). Yi, a young woman attached to one of the seventeen production brigades, had received one year of training previously and had returned to the commune hospital for three months of additional training. Her original year of medical education had included the study of pharmacology, physiology and physical hygiene, minimal amounts of anatomy, and the diagnosis of common diseases. Yi was currently learning to give injections, to treat minor injury and trauma, and to improve her diagnostic skill.

Her six-day work week included three days in health work and three days in agricultural labor, but some of this time was devoted to production brigade medicinal herb growing. Her responsibilities included health education (primarily personal hygiene) and this is accomplished, she said, during her work breaks in the field, at brigade meetings, and when she is giving treatment. She is considered to be on 24-hour duty and also makes regular house visits. We were told that her training and work were what is conventionally done by BFDs at 5th May.

The 5th May Commune was clearly a productive and wealthy commune by Chinese standards. Its economy was diversified and included vegetables and rice production, the raising of pigs, chickens, and rabbits and a stock farm that sends 800,000 kilos of fresh milk to the Shenyang market. It also had a mechanized chicken processing plant and a large pool of equipment. It was currently engaged in a project to bring running water to all the commune households. The 5th May Commune provided both primary- and middle-school education to all children and there were numerous other signs of a well-established commune. However, when asked if the 5th May would soon be able to afford full-time Barefoot Doctors, that is to release them from all agricultural responsibilities, the response was "No," it was unlikely that any agricultural manpower could be spared for full-time medical work in the next three to five years. Even plans for further mechanization of farm work could not permit any additional released time. Other agricultural needs would take priority over full-time medical work. Up to this time no 5th May Commune BFDs had taken certification exams.

KaiAn Commune: Rural BFD (Models One, Two, and Three). A visit to a distant rural commune some 60 kilometers from the major northern city of Chang Chun provided the opportunity to see a BFD program in a remote area and at a different level of rural health care delivery (Study Journal 1979:156–192). KaiAn Commune, with a population of 29,782, supports a district commune hospital serving its own needs and those of five or six other communes.

We have previously discussed 5th May Commune as having Barefoot Doctors representative of Model Three, and for contrast it appears that KaiAn Commune utilizes all three models of training and practice of BFDs.

Model One Barefoot Doctors are trained at the local level by district hospital physicians who rotate to the commune production teams and teach Barefoot Doctors exclusively through practical work. Model Two Barefoot Doctors are sent to the Commune District Hospital for training. Within the last ten years, KaiAn Commune has trained 180 Barefoot Doctors at this level. Model Three Barefoot Doctors are sent to the county or city hospital for initial and advanced training. Within the last ten years, KaiAn has had 400 Barefoot Doctors receive training at this advanced level.

Of the thirty-nine Barefoot Doctors presently employed in the KaiAn Commune Clinic, sixteen were trained at a city or county hospital at the advanced Model Three level. The remaining twenty-three were trained at either the commune hospital or by a mobile medical team, either at Model One or Two levels. We interviewed one Barefoot Doctor who appears to exemplify Model Three typology in that her initial training was a total of one year in length and involved six months at the county hospital level, four months in KaiAn Commune Clinic, and two months at the city medical center. Her curriculum throughout involved pediatrics, maternity care, internal medicine, surgery, and Chinese herbs.

Within the KaiAn Commune Clinic, medical practice of Model One BFD was described as generally involving the following:

1. Treatment emphasizes preventive work rather than curative techniques. Mass campaigns for prevention, early diagnosis, and treatment to protect the labor force and encourage production were listed as priorities for this level of practitioner. Since 1971, because of the success of this level of intervention, diphtheria, encephalitis, whooping cough, measles, scarlet fever, and diarrhea have been brought under control.

2. The preventive work also involves family planning by instructing the peasants in birth control during group meetings and using the commune broadcasting system, which has

speakers placed throughout the commune. All BFDs were engaged in agricultural work and none had taken exams.

Rural-Urban Comparison. A number of important observations can be made as we contrast the BFDs on a wealthy suburban commune (5th May) and a distant rural commune (KaiAn). The 5th May's "typical" BFD has Model Three training that is *less* medically sophisticated than the Model Three BFD at the distant commune. The 5th May BFD's job description is exclusively prevention and health education but she is now improving her primary care skills. The distant rural commune emphasizes BFDs at all levels of development and more delineated jobs. Model Ones work exclusively at prevention. Model Threes are called on to do much more medically advanced work. Further, the wealthiest commune sees no early prospect for BFDs to become full-time BFDs. Of course, their need for that is less because they have easy access to fully trained physicians in the nearby city.

This substantiates all the earlier observations concerning the variability of BFD training, skills, and what they are called on to do. Table 1.2 gathers together a review of much of the BFD literature and adds our 1979 material. The one consistent piece of information in all reports is BFD/population ratios, and an analysis of these does reflect on variability in terms of how many workers can be spared for health work and, by implication, what they will be called upon to do.

One is also tempted to see if there are changes over time and Table 1.2 has been arranged chronologically in terms of when reports appeared in the literature. No patterns of change emerge between 1971 and 1979 as far as these limited ratios are concerned.

BFD/Population Ratios. According to Tsui (1979:87), the national goal is one BFD for every 500 in the population. Current information states that there are 1.5 million Barefoot Doctors. Using a population figure of 900 million, we have calculated a national ratio of about 1:650. This is close to a recently released official figure claiming a mean of 1:616. We have taken Table 1.2 and reorganized it according to proximity to major urban area (Table 1.3). Some interesting differences reveal themselves. Beijing ratios are strikingly lower than all other cities. We may assume this reflects two things: the communes visited were "suburban" and therefore wealthier and with good access to city facilities, and that there would be greater incentives to fulfill policy so close to the capitol. The 5th May Commune, which our group visited, is positively identified as a "wealthy" suburban commune and its ratio is at least twice as high as other reports of communes in the Shenyang region. Obviously this is limited material, but it clearly reflects wide disparities around the country ranging from 1:207 to 1:1623, and we can see that geographic location is at least one meaningful correlate of existing ratios.

BFD Training Programs

Nong An County Hospital: Rural Training. The Nong An County Hospital, located in a town of 96,000, has an attached medical school that trains nurses and also offers a Barefoot Doctor training program (Study Journal 1969:178–185). In existence since 1972, it has trained 400 of these paramedics in six-month training courses. Apparently, a small number go on to the medical college: in 1978, four of the class were admitted to advanced medical training. The total number of Barefoot Doctors now in the county is 1,200, the best of which were sent to this county-level hospital training program. Physicians from the county hospital also go to the commune district centers (such as KaiAn Commune) to give periodic lectures to local Barefoot Doctors.

The director of Nong An Hospital, who was our host, said that those few who get advanced training will ". . . no longer be Barefoot Doctors but doctors," and therefore will work in medical care full-time. However, he also described the new national policy that by 1985 all Barefoot Doctors would be trained up to the expertise of middle-level-school doctors and be able to treat "common disease."

County hospitals are an important link in Barefoot Doctor training. It is worth noting that Nong An's Medical School has provided[4] additional training for one-third of the county's paramedics.

As for the educational content of the county BFD training, there was a very heavy emphasis on Traditional herbal medicines and the extensive utilization of Traditional techniques like acupuncture. Further, the hospital had a large herbal garden used to supply the hospital and to educate BFDs.

Beijing Municipal General Hospital: Urban Training. We were able to gather a small amount of information about the involvement of urban facilities in the BFD program (Study Journal 1979:189–213). The Beijing hospital system has a rural rotation dispatch team involved in training Barefoot Doctors in a 27-month program similar to the Model Three Barefoot Training discussed earlier. Fifteen months of the training is accrued training and occurs in the commune-level clinics. Specifically, in the Beijing area rotation program, the team is composed of western and Traditional physicians and one to three well-trained Barefoot Doctors. This team rotates to rural areas for a period of one year. When asked about specifics of the training program, an official of the Tong Ren Branch Hospital indicated the following:

(1) All Barefoot Doctors have one year of initial training followed by

(2) five months per year of additional training over a three-year period for a total of twenty-seven months of training;

(3) the additional accrued fifteen months of training beyond the initial one year will occur in the commune clinics, will involve upgrading the diagnostic and operation skills of Barefoot Doctors and will be given by the rural dispatch team from Tong Ren Branch Hospital.

The official from Tong Ren also indicated that other programs vary greatly in the length of Barefoot Doctor training and that there is not uniformity throughout China in this training.

Rural-Urban Education Comparison. Comparing the two BFD educational programs, the county hospital program, which according to policy statements is to do the bulk of BFD upgrading, is actively functioning for its county BFDs and has trained a third of them at the Model Three level. However, their training program reflects their own heavy reliance on Traditional approaches. This suggests less adequately prepared BFDs called on to perform at a higher level of skill. It is worth observing that they interpret the new national policy to mean that all BFDs will become full-time higher level physicians. We would suggest that this reflects their greater need for such personnel. The BFD training program based in Beijing appears to be much more rigorous and better organized, and to be putting a major emphasis on western medicine. Furthermore, their training program is serving the counties in the Beijing area, thereby bringing more elaborate BFD training to communes with greater access to urban facilities.

We have extrapolated from our training program material to structure Table 1.4, which refers back to our suburban and rural communes. It is clear that the rural commune with fewer BFDs trained in a county hospital program asks for the most complex medical work. It also make the important point that a single commune is utilizing BFDs trained and performing on various levels.

Keeping the CMA briefing in mind, several observations can be made about the BFD policy in action at the grass roots level of the health care system in 1979. The contradiction in training and tasks is reflected. The assertion that BFDs will remain part-time is corroborated. The mixture of medical, prevention, and health education responsibilities is shown. However, the field information suggests a process of differentiation taking place among BFDs so that some will indeed remain part-time Model One BFDs, while others are slowly filtering up into another rank (assistant doctor) in China's medical manpower pool. There is no indication that the examinations for certification have yet taken place. The material suggests, however, the new BFD policy at an early normative stage with little indication of action on the grass roots level but small hints of future difficulties in implementing full-time medical work for BFDs.

The Barefoot Doctor Situation in 1981

Policy Statements. Between 1979 and 1981, a review of *Mainland China Press* (January 1981; March 1981; September 1981) revealed several important policy statements that elaborated on the push for BFD upgrading that we first heard about at the CMA briefing. These included important indications of central government subsidies to upgrade the rural health care system targeting one-third of the county hospitals, the granting of special certificates of practice to BFDs who pass the competency exams and refresher courses to those who fail. Special categories of BFDs, however, are to be granted certificates without taking a written exam: (1) those who have been BFDs since 1966 and have, therefore, extensive practical experience; (2) those with over one year of training in a provincial or higher level hospital; (3) those already in possession of a medium-grade or higher medical school certificate. In point of fact, the Ministry of Health stated that by September 1981, one-third of the 1.5 million BFDs have obtained village (or county) doctor certificates.[5] (There is no way of knowing how many of them did it by having these special characteristics.)

The issue of pay for the BFDs has also been discussed in some detail by the Ministry of Health. Official policy is that certificated BFDs are to be full-time and paid the same salary as local school teachers. Those in the process of "training up" are to get the usual work points plus a subsidy. The subsidy is to address complaints by BFDs that their work loads do not permit them to keep pace with the rising income of their fellow workers with private plots. Apparently this issue and the refusal of some localities to adjust BFD pay has caused a number to leave their medical work.

BFDs are to move more exclusively toward clinical work. Finally, the most recent policy states that the assessment, training, certification, and transfer of BFDs will be the exclusive responsibility of the county public health bureaus who will also manage government subsidies for the program.

Observations. On our second visit, both rural and suburban communes were visited including several days in Ye County,[6] a successful agricultural area with some of the best health statistics in the PRC. Our 1979 material has been rendered in some detail focusing on training, responsibilities, and model level of various BFDs. All of this kind of information and more has been rendered in chart form for the 1981 material (Study Journal 1981) (Table 1.5).

Discussion. Noteworthy in the 1981 material is that while there is considerably more continuing education in the urban locations, the rural BFDs are called on to do somewhat more sophisticated medical work. Nowhere is there any indication of heavier emphasis or movement toward clinical work. All the BFDs in both suburban and rural locations have been studying for exams, which according to our information, appears to be given on two levels—an initial exam perhaps eliciting a "BFD certificate" and a higher-level exam to obtain the country doctor certificate. Only a handful of the urban BFDs have attained this latter status; the rest are on the initial exam level. Only in suburban areas were we able to find a full-time BFD. All others still do agricultural work. And nowhere is a BFD being paid a salary (although subsidies are given in suburban Shanghai). Everywhere we went BFDs are improving knowledge and skills using continuing education at county hospitals and medical schools and, as mentioned in one commune, a special three-times-a-week (four-year) television course.

Conclusions

By juxtaposing observations of BFDs in 1979 and 1981, we can garner hints of evolving BFD policy and slowly evolving implementation of that policy. We can also note continuing differences around the country. There is, however, growing consistency in job responsibilities between rural and suburban areas. The rural areas all appear to be behind in length of training, while still asking more of their BFDs. The issue of full-time and salaried status for BFDs is certainly not resolved.

In several communes we were told that details of the new BFD policy were being studied and discussed. But even the most affluent communes we visited in suburban Shanghai and rural Ye county were not even contemplating full-time medical work and salaries for their BFDs. This issue will be problematic for some time to come. The central government now stands behind a normative policy that continues to be vulnerable to local economic exigencies, raising expectations that will be deferentially met. The major differences in the two-year period between the 1979 and 1981 visits is that the upgrading process is found everywhere in a centrally motivated push to improve the quality of care that BFDs provide. The government is addressing the central criticism of BFDs that emerged in the 1970s.

Mao's need to better serve the rural masses almost twenty years after the Revolution created a new medical manpower category, a creative innovation that would accomplish a number of goals in one stroke. The major goal was to overcome the continuing rural maldistribution of physicians in the PRC. The health worker created, however, was not a physician, although the label "doctor" was utilized. The Barefoot Doctor was picked differently, trained differently, paid differently, and functions differently than the conventional professional physician.

The most current national health policy is taking another innovative step. The Barefoot Doctor is now to be professionalized. To move the Barefoot Doctor toward increased professionalization is perhaps just as daring as Mao's original Barefoot Doctor plan. It is part of the commitment to modernization of the current leadership and an example of the professionalization process taking place in other segments of the labor force as well. It also reflects the general return to power and dominance of the professionals and experts. There is some irony here as a political creation of the 1960s, brought to life outside the bounds of professional medical models and control, now moves back precisely toward that model and its influence.

The process of professionalization is well-known (Friedson 1970) from a sociological perspective. If extensive numbers of Barefoot Doctors receive additional education commensurate with that of assistant doctors, then one might predict that some of them will insist on moving more to curative services, to some status-distancing from their patients, and to closer identification with professional medical norms and values. This may mean that some of the laudable features of the earlier policy will give way, in the name of improved quality of health care, to professionalization and the characteristics that typify it.

The unevenness in both quality and quantity of Barefoot Doctors around the country will no doubt slow the professionalization process. As has been pointed out and substantiated, variability will continue to be related to economic and geographic factors unless there is long-term central government subsidy to the program. Barefoot Doctors continue to be vulnerable to the exigencies of agricultural output and local conditions.

It was only because of Mao's boldness that the nation has been able to increase its medical manpower pool and improve (but by no means balance) distribution. The BFD program, albeit in new garb, may be the one major Maoist policy to survive and be strengthened under the new regime. Mao proclaimed a policy counter to general professional models that emphasize expertise first for the delivery of medical care. He could only implement such a nonprofessional program where professional doctors were relatively weak and lacked the political power to resist such a threat to their control of medical knowledge and health care delivery. It is also clear that this strategy has its serious problems, discovered when one looks beyond stated policy and examines the realities of grass roots implementation.

A road to professionalization has been opened for China's Bareoot Doctors. How well it is paved, how well traveled it will be, and where it will lead remain unclear. Considerable research will be needed to understand better how Mao's original creation takes care of China's doctor shortage and maldistribution (Blendon 1979:1457). If Bareoot Doctors remain in place and receive increased training to bring them uniformly up to the level of primary care physicians by western standards, then Mao's political strategy of 1965 will provide an unusual model for the chronic problem of physician shortages and maldistribution in rural areas, faced by many other nations' health care systems. The important point to note however, is that this is quite a different strategy from the creation of a permanent cadre of paraprofessionals to deliver care.

NOTES

1. Like much material collected to date in the PRC, this is based on an accumulated period of about thirty-four days and involves half-day visits to various facilities in three different regions of the country. The authors were both in China in 1979; Rosenthal returned in 1981.

2. The 23 June 1980 issue of the *Beijing Review* carries an article on this subject noting that Deng Xiaoping, when he was in charge of the work of the State Council in 1975, remarked graphically that "Barefoot Doctors should eventually wear shoes . . . expressing the hope that they would increase their medical knowledge and raise their professional

proficiency." This was apparently the impetus for developing the new policy.

3. Unger (1980:45), in an article on current trends in PRC higher education, makes the provocative observation that BFDs who are able to go on to university medical education may often be city youth who have been sent down to the countryside. Being chosen BFD may provide a route back to university education.

4. Only a very small fraction of Nong An BFDs have continued on for university medical school. Let us assume that the four who did so in 1978 represent the annual figures (a liberal assumption); therefore in eight years this equals thirty-two (0.2 percent) of the total number of Barefoot Doctors.

5. Some specific figures on certification have appeared in the *Mainland China Press*. Guangdong Province: started 1978; 80 percent of BFDs received further training; of these 70,000 BFDs, 84 percent got certification after exams. Jiangsu Province: seventy-five counties, seventy-three have conducted BFD exams, 76 percent BFDs obtained certification. Qinghai Province (rural and pastoral areas) had 800 BFDs; 60 percent reached village doctor level. (Source: *New China News Agency*; Hua Chi, 3 September 1981).

6. Ye Hsein (county) in Shandong Province (pop: 827,000 with 94 percent in agricultural work) has a 1980 infant mortality rate of 11.7/1,000, life expectancy rates of seventy-two for males and seventy-seven for females; leading causes of death are stroke and heart disease. Its BFD/Population ratio is 1:374, well below the national average. It is an impressive model of health accomplishments that do not depend on industrialization.

TABLE 1.1
Development of Medical Manpower in the PRC

	1966[a]	1979[b]	1981[c]
Physicians	157,500	395,000[d]	
Assistant doctors	179,000	435,000[d]	960,000 (est.)
Traditional doctors		423,000	
Medical assistants			
Midwives	44,000		
Nurses	193,000	421,000	
Dentists	31,500		
Pharmacists	21,000		
Junior pharmacists	52,000		
Technical assistants			
Laboratory			
technicans	52,000		
Barefoot Doctors		1,575,000[d]	1,050,000 (est.)
Health aides		4,200,000	

a   Adapted from: Cheny, Chu-Yuan, "Health Manpower: Growth and Distribution" in Myron Wegman, editor, Public Health in the PRC. New York: The Macy Foundation, 1973, Pp. 139-57. And Taylor, Carl, "Report of a Trip to China . . ." Johns Hopkins School of Public Health, 1980.

b   From: Chen, Pi-Chao, "Population Policy and the Rural Health System in China." World Bank Monograph, May 1981.

c   From: Interview with Minister of Health, New China News Agency; Hua Chi 20, 3 September 1981.

d   Current policy goal by 1985.

TABLE 1.2
Barefoot Doctor Distribution in the People's Republic of China: A Summary of Authors from 1971 to 1981

Year	Area	Population	BFD/Population Ratio	Proximity to Urban Area	Author and source of Information
1971	Mai Chia Wu Production Team	251	1:126	Near Hangchow	Sidel, V.W. Serve the People, 1973
1971	Double North Production Team	500	1:250	Outside Peking	Sidel, V.W. IJHS, 2(3), 1972
1971	Sing Sing Production Brigade	1,850	1:463	Outside Shanghai	Sidel, V.W. SA 230(4) April 1974
1971	Taipingchaio Production Brigade	2,900	1:207	Near Peking on main bus line	Sidel, V.W. Serve the People, 1973
1971	Taichai Commune	10,000	1:303	Shansi Province; 48 km/30 mi to Yu-tzu	-
1971	Double Bridge Commune	38,000	1:241	Outside Peking	Sidel, V.W. IJHS, 2(3), 1972, p. 391
1971	10 Shanghai communes	4 million	1:519	Entire Shanghai rural area	Sidel, V.W. IJHS, 2(3), 1972
1973	4 Seasons	22,000	1:710	Near Hangchow	Li, Victor. Stanford Law Review, 2, 1975
	Evergreen Commune	21,890	1:706	Near Hangchow	New, Peter. Human Organization, 34(3), 1975
		28,900	1:903	Near Hangchow	Wang, Virginia. IJHS, 5(30), 1975
1973	July One Commune	16,963	1:514	Near Shanghai	New, Peter. Human Organization, 34(3), 1975
1973	August One Commune	20,853	1:802	Near Shenyang	New, Peter. Ekistics, 226, 1974
		21,000	1:808	Near Shenyang	Wang, Virginia. IJHS, 5(30), 1975
		28,053	1:1078	Near Shenyang	New, Peter. Human Organization, 34(3), 1975
1973	Nan-Ying Commune	27,000	1:482	Near Shanghai	
1973	Tsao-ying Village Commune	70,000	1:1458	Near Shanghai	-
1973	Mei Chai Commune	10,440	1:208	Near Hangchow, 7.2 km/4.5 mi	-
1974	Shin Hua Commune	63,600	1:1590	Outside Canton	McKinnon, New England J. Med., 13 March 1974
1974	#1 Commune	14,807	1:617	No locations indicated	Kleinman & Mechanic, JNMD, 1979
1975	#2 Commune	13,514	1:1229		-
1975	#3 Commune	18,158	1:256		-
1975	#4 Commune	43,129	1:1797		-
1976	#5 Commune	15,230	1:1269		-
1976	#6 Commune	19,481	1:1623		-
1976	#7 Commune	8,396	1:700		-
1976	#8 Commune	12,837	1:1283		-
1976	#9 Commune	1,978	1:659		-
1976	#10 Commune	12,999	1:542		-
1976	#11 Commune	17,694	1:492		-

Year	Area	Population	BFD/ Population Ratio	Proximity to Urban Area	Author and source of Information
1977	Heng County	780,000	1:600	In Kwangsi Province	Mechanic & Kleinman, 1978
1977	San Yang Commune	22,900	1:636	240 km to Changsa (more rural)	"
1978	Doushan Commune	57,934	1:689	30 km SW of Taicheng. Canton area	Tsui, 1979
1978	Huancheng Commune	60,000	1:706	Close to Huicheng 41.6 km/26 mi (Canton area)	"
1978	Shaanxi Province	26 million	1:260		Rogers, Rural Health in the PRC, 1980
1978	Hunan Province	48 million	1:371		"
1978	Miyun County	380,000	1:220	Beijing Municipality	"
1978	Heng County	780,000	1:569	Guangxi Autonomous Region	"
1978	Xinhui County	830,000	1:616	Guangdong Province	"
1978	Henanzhai Commune	21,000	1:191	Miyun County	"
1978	Dazhai Commune	11,600	1:223	Xiyang County	"
1978	Luancun Commune	17,430	1:405	Chang'an County Shaanxi Province	"
1978	Chuanshan Commune	18,600	1:413	(near Guilin) Guangxi Autonomous Region	"
1978	Taoxu Commune	56,923	1:513	Heng County Guangxi Autonomous Region	"
1979	Nong An County	960,000	1:800	60 km NW of Chang Chun	Study Journals, 1979
1979	Kaian Commune	29,782	1:764	33 km to Chang Chun	"
1979	5th May People's Commune	39,000	1:433	30 km to Nong An County Suburban Shenyang	"
1981	Ye County	827,500	1:374	Shandong Province	Study Journals, 1981

Note: The variable, geographic location, which means proximity to a large urban environment, has to be understood within the context of Chinese society. For example, the 1979 Study Tour was told that Kaian Commune was a "distant rural" setting. Reference to a reliable map when we returned to the States revealed that Kaian is 33 km from the major city of Chang Chun (population 1.5 million). This barely seems remote by American standards. Perhaps this was merely a case of the guide's attempt to placate our request to visit a distant rural area. Or perhaps it reflects limited transportation and the concept of distance in a primarily agricultural nation.

TABLE 1.3
Proximity to Cities and BFD-Population Ratios (Selected Figures)

Canton	Hangchow	Beijing	Shanghai	Shanyang	Ye County (deviant case)
1:1590	1:126	1:207	1:463	1:433	1:374
1:706	1:208	1:241	1:482	1:802	
1:689	1:706	1:250	1:514	1:808	
	1:710	1:220	1:1458	1:1078	
	1:903	1:191	1:1519		
			(combines ten communes)		

City	Population	Mean	Median
Beijing	7.570 million (one-half in suburban countryside)	1:221	1:241
Hangchow	980,000	1:611	1:706
Shanghai	10.8 million (5.2 million in suburban countryside)	1:729	1:514
Shenyang	3 million (including suburban countryside)	1:896	1:802

1980 National Mean: 1:616
National Goal: 1:500

Lowest: 1:207
Highest: 1:1623
Overall mean: 1:650
Overall median: 1:514

Sources: PRC State Statistical Bureau, 1980 (from Chen 1980); Tsui, 1979.

TABLE 1.4
Geographical Location and Medical Practice Description

	Rural (KaiAn, rural Chang Chun)	Suburban (5th May Commune, Suburban Shenyang)
Production brigade clinic	Model One and Two BFD; Model Three as supervisor and trainer of lower level health workers	Model One BFD
Commune Hospital	Traditional and western doctors secondary-level doctors Model 3 BFD	Model Two and Three BFD
	less referrals	more referrals
	Barefoot Doctors-Population Ratio 764:1	Barefoot Doctors-Population Ratio 433:1
	higher level practice at lower tier	lower level practice at higher tier

Source: Study Journal 1979.

TABLE 1.5
BFD Information—1981

Commune and Other	Preliminary Training	Continuing Education	Responsibility	Compensation	No. BFD Full- or Part-Time	Current Status
Malu Suburban Shanghai (all at production brigade level)	3 months in county hospital medical school	2-3 years in county hospital	Population planning ante/ post natal care. first aide Model 1.2	Workpoints and subsidies	Still have agricultural responsibilities 3/brigade. 48 total (32 practicing at least 10 years)	All have taken county exam; preparing to take certification exam on city level in fall; 10 have CDC
Dong Fang Production Brigade, suburban Canton	3 months	1-2 years in county hospital	Immunizations, colds, bronchitis, intestinal disease. after-hospital care. prevention campaigns Model 1.2	Workpoints	8 Full-time	1 has BFD certificate (1st phase of exams)
Guo Xi Rural Ye County	3-6 months in county hospital medical school	1 year in commune hospital	Population planning ante/ post natal care. first aide, common illness Model 1.2.3	Workpoints	Still have agricultural responsibilities 75 in 23 PB clinics	61 have BFD certificates
Guo Xi Production Brigades #1 and 2	County hospital			Workpoints[a]	3/clinic	BFD certificate
Ye County (general info)	6 months in county hospital medical school	1 year in commune hospital	Campaigns, social sanitation, stitching wounds, cutting tumors Model 1.2.3	Workpoints	Still have agricultural responsibilities 2,212	All have taken exam; 10% failed-- getting more training; 2,212 BFD certificate; none country doctor certificate

[a] A BFD in Guo Xi Production Brigade Clinic #1 gave us a breakdown of workpoints last year: workpoints = 3,600, 10 workpoints = 2 yuan = 360 yuan.
Source: Study Journal 1981.

REFERENCES

Beijing Review
  1980 23 June
Beijing Xinhua
  1981 Beijing Xinhua Domestic Service in Chinese; 070 GMT
    Survey of Mainland China Press Magazines, January
    1981, 24 March 1981; 3 September 1981.
Blendon, R. J.
  1979 Can China's Health Care Be Transplanted Without
    China's Economic Policies? New England Journal of
    Medicine 300:1453–458.
Chen, Peter
  1981 Population Policy and the Rural Health System in
    China. Report to the World Bank.
Cheng, C.
  1973 Health Manpower: Growth and Distribution. In Public
    Health in the People's Republic of China. M. E. Wegman
    et al., eds. Pp. 139–157. New York: Josiah Macy,
    Jr. Foundation.
Friedson, E.
  1970 The Profession of Medicine. New York: Dodd, Mead.
Ginzberg, E.
  1978 Health, Manpower and Health Policy. New York:
    Universe Books.
Hsu, R.
  1974 The Barefoot Doctor of the People's Republic of China.
    New England Journal of Medicine 291:124–127.
Kleinman, A., and D. Mechanic
  1979 Some Observations of Mental Illness and Its Treatment
    in the People's Republic of China. The Journal of Nervous
    and Mental Disease 167:267–274.
Lampton, D. M.
  1977 The Politics of Medicine in China. Boulder, Colo.:
    Westview Press.
  1978 Performance and the Chinese Political System: A
    Preliminary Assessment of Education and Health Policies.
    China Quarterly 75:509–539.
  1978 Development and Health Care: Is China's Medical
    Programme Exportable? World Development 6:621–630.

Li, V. H.
1975 Politics and Health Care in China: The Barefoot Doctors. Stanford Law Review 27:827–840.
Lucas, Anelisa
1980 Changing Medical Models in China: Organizational Options or Obstacles? China Quarterly: September 1980.
McKinnon, J.
1974 A Glimpse of Medicine in China. New Zealand Medical Journal 79:13, March.
Mechanic, D., and A. Kleinman
1978 The Organization, Delivery and Financing of Rural Care in the People's Republic of China. Research and Analytic Report Series No. 10. University of Wisconsin, Madison.
New China Monthly
1950 The Correct Direction in People's Health Work. 13:166.
New, P. K.
1974 Barefoot Doctors and Health Care in the People's Republic of China. Ekistics 2:220–224.
1975 The Links between Health and the Political Structure in New China. Human Organization 34:237–251.
Rifkin, S. B.
1973 Health Care for Rural Areas. In Medicine and Public Health in the People's Republic of China. J. R. Quinn, ed. U. S. Department of Health, Education and Welfare.
Rogers, E. M.
1980 Barefoot Doctors. In Rural Health in the People's Republic of China. Committee on Scholarly Communication with the People's Republic of China. NIH Publication No. 81–2124. November 1981.
Sidel, V. W.
1972 The Barefoot Doctors of the People's Republic of China. New England Journal of Medicine 286:1292–1300.
1972 Some Observations on the Organization of Health Care in the People's Republic of China. International Journal of Health Services 2:385–395.
Sidel, V. W., and R. Sidel
1973 Serve the People: Observations on Medicine in the People's Republic of China. New York: Josiah Macy, Jr. Foundation.

1974 The Delivery of Medical Care in China. Scientific American 230:19–27.

Study Group Journals

1979 Journal of the University of Michigan-Dearborn/ Michigan State University Health Care Study Tour. (Available upon request from Professor Rosenthal).

1981 Journal of the University of Michigan-Dearborn/ Michigan State University Health Care Study Tour. (Available upon request from Professor Rosenthal).

Taylor, C. E.

1980 Report of a Trip to China . . . 31 October – 25 November 1980. Department of International Health, The Johns Hopkins University, School of Hygiene and Public Health.

Tsui, W.

1979 Regionalization and Accessibility of Rural Health Services in the People's Republic of China: A Comparative Case Study of the Huancheng and Doushan Communes. Masters thesis submitted to the Chinese University of Hong Kong (under supervision of Professor Rance P. L. Lee).

Unger, J.

1980 The Chinese Controversy Over Higher Education. Pacific Affairs 53:29–47.

Wang, V. L.

1975 Training of the Barefoot Doctor in the People's Republic of China. International Journal of Health Services 5:476– 486.

2
POLITICAL PROCESS AND THE INTEGRATION OF TRADITIONAL AND WESTERN MEDICINE IN THE PEOPLE'S REPUBLIC OF CHINA

INTRODUCTION

On the second floor of China Medical University Hospital in Shenyang is a small room with unique medical decor. The decorations are for the edification of visiting foreign friends. Half of a wall is handsomely lettered with the titles of medical conditions the hospital treats with Traditional herbs. Beneath each title is a list of symptomatology, the herbal prescription, the number of cases treated with success rates. The conditions are essentially 'acute abdomines' and include appendicitis, intestinal obstructions, gastric perforation, pancreatis and gall stones. There is a featured display of this latter disease to which the visitor's attention is directed: a long table covered with several dozen Petrie dishes. Each holds a small collection of gall stones that range in size from one-half to 4 cm. The attending doctor relates that various patients 'passed' these stones aided by herbal medicines that enlarged the ducts sufficiently for this to occur. Thus, in a number of cases, gall bladder removal was avoided saving the patient the risks of surgery and its debilitating recovery period.

The display also reflects an economical utilization of resources in a country of limited means. It typifies the variety of ways the health care system of the People's Republic of

Reprinted with permission from Social Science and Medicine Vol. 15A, 1981, Pergamon Press, Ltd.

China has responded to Chairman Mao's 1950 dictum to integrate Traditional Chinese medicine with western medicine. The People's Republic of China, he declared, would create a new medicine and make a significant contribution to world culture.

In August of 1979, during a health care study tour of the People's Republic we visited some seventeen different health facilities and talked to several dozen health workers. These ranged from neighborhood Red Medical workers in Beijing to Barefoot Doctors in the distant rural commune of KaiAn north of Chang Chun. We toured simple health stations as well as a teaching hospital doing advanced research. A subject of particular interest to us was the attempt to integrate Traditional Chinese and western medicine.

Our attention to this subject had been stimulated by reports of earlier visitors and enthusiasts who described the integration in glowing terms and held it up as a model of appropriate and desirable utilization of cultural traditions (Horn 1969; Sidel 1973). Our extensive material reflects the wealth of information we were able to obtain on this as well as other characteristics of the health system. This information was not gathered under ideal research circumstances and one must be cautious about generalizability.[1] However, it is extensive enough to permit a contribution to the on-going discussion of this unique experiment in the Chinese system.

A UNIQUE EXPERIMENT IN MEDICAL HISTORY

In July 1950, shortly after the revolutionary success of the Chinese Communist Party, and the Liberation of 1949, the First National Health Conference on Public Health was being held in Beijing. Chairman Mao addressed that conference and laid out the four principles that were to shape, and continue to shape, the health care system of the People's Republic of China (Crozier 1965): (1) medicine must serve the masses; (2) put prevention first; (3) health work should utilize mass campaigns; (4) integrate Chinese Traditional and western medicine.

This was not the first time Chairman Mao had made a public pronouncement on the utilization of Chung-i (Traditional Chinese Medicine). Nor was this a new issue in modern

Chinese society. The fate of the old tradition had been a social and intellectual issue for a number of decades, back actually to the Ching dynasty, the last of the Emperors. At issue was the usefulness and status of a 2000-year-old medical tradition that encompassed a fully articulated theory, a complex approach to medical diagnosis and a repertoire of treatment techniques. For example, an important element in its theoretical super-structure is the concept of Yin and Yang, hypothesized polar-opposite forces in the body that have to remain in harmony for the maintenance of personal health. Among its diagnostic tech-niques is the recognition of twelve different body pulse systems which can be utilized in the recognition of disease and illness. And among its treatment techniques are acupuncture, herbal remedies, moxibustion, cupping, massage and unique approaches to bone fracture. It claims efficaciousness on the basis of hundreds of years of clinical experience. It is the longest-lived medical tradition in human history, a complex component of the old Confucian culture. By the turn of the century, it was on its way to historical oblivion and consign-ment to the museum of medical oddities, victim to the rising dominance of western bio-medical science although it still had a pervasive rural following.

Mao Tse-tung's political and economic interest in preserving Chung-i raised an old issue to new heights. He cast its future into the political arena, both in terms of the on-going evolution of national health policy and in terms of the local, day-to-day delivery of health care in the People's Republic of China. Rescued from repeated attacks in the face of the modern embrace of science, Mao's directive launched a unique endeavor in world-wide health care delivery. What is its history? What has been the political fate of Mao's policy declaration in 1950? What does 'integration' look like in prac-tical terms today? What can be said about the future of Chung-i, particularly in the face of China's current, renewed commitment to modernization?

A look at the literature and a description of what the writer saw and heard may provide some tentative answers to these questions. A review of previous analyses suggests that Croizier, more than any other American scholar, has examined the issue of Traditional medicine in Chinese political and intel-lectual life in greatest depth (Croizier 1968).

PRE-LIBERATION CCP STANCE ON TRADITIONAL MEDICINE

Croizier points out that early Chinese Communist Party (CCP) writing reflected considerable antipathy to Chung-i. In a 1915 issue of *Call to Youth*, this tradition was held up as the epitome of feudalism in old Chinese culture (Croizier 1968). It was ridiculed as superstitious, irrational and backward—all that the Communists wanted to destroy in their commitment to rebuilding a modern, progressive China. Croizier describes this ridicule as common in party literature which also reflects the party's dedication to modern sciences as the symbol of progress. During Nanking government debates on the future of Traditional medicine, Communist leaders argued that it was a primitive, unscientific stage of medical development. The one major voice of support came from right-wing Nationalists who argued for its preservation (Croizier 1968).

The Civil War, however, found the CCP dealing with the issue on more pragmatic terms. During the Kiangsi Soviet and the years in Yenan, practical problems of health and medical care were confronted. Kiangsi, the first area of Communist domination, produced an attempt to utilize local herbs as a substitute for western medicines made scarce because of the Nationalist blockade. However, modern medical approaches and public hygiene measures were instituted where possible. In Yenan, primitive factories produced herbal and simple medicines and the 'less harmful' Traditional doctors were 'tolerated'. But at the same time the *Army Medical Journal* expressed considerable criticism of Traditional medicine while recognizing the empirical value of selected herbs.

During the Civil War and the Japanese blockades, it is significant to note that one of the great revolutionary heroes to emerge was Dr Norman Bethune. He was a Canadian physician whose battlefield surgical feats became part of Communist lore (Gordon 1952). He was also a physician very much in the western mode.

The first official CCP pronouncement of what might be considered a protopolicy on Traditional medicine came during the 1944 Border Area Conference on Culture and Education.

Here Mao spoke about uniting the two medicines and 'improving' the Traditional with science. He is quoted as saying:

> To surrender to the old style is wrong; to abolish or discard is wrong; our responsibility is to unite those of the old style that can be used and to help, stimulate and reform them (Croizier 1968).

He exhorts western-trained physicians to improve Chung-i and to form a 'United Front' of the new and old style medicine. He calls for organizing, up-grading and utilizing Traditional doctors to 'meet critical needs'. Mao at this time publicly sanctions the use of the old medicine as part of a larger strategy to deal with the massive health problems of the nation. These ideas were echoed at the 1950 First National Conference on Public Health which took place a year after Liberation. Western-style doctors were urged to take major responsibility in bringing the old medicine into the modern medical mainstream.

Croizier is able to provide information about implementation of the policy after the 1950 Conference. One of the first steps was to break down the secrecy and private practice of the individual Traditional doctors. They were now encouraged to join group practice clinics, formed primarily in rural areas. Short courses in modern medicine were established for these doctors to broaden their medical knowledge.

In 1954 and 1955, as prelude to the Great Leap, quite another approach developed. The Party became much more actively involved in the promotion of the integration as part of a larger effort to assert party control over the educated professionals of the country. As part of the 'Red versus Expert' battle, because of the 'unwillingness' of physicians to be guided by party ideology and the accusation that they were clinging to bourgeois thinking, massive criticism of western-trained doctors was carried out. This included the insistence that they engage in self-criticism of their conservative attitudes and their continuing skepticism and ridicule of Traditional medicine. It included a strong push for them to engage in their own systematic study of the Tradition.

There also developed an articulation of cultural pride in past accomplishments and a wave of publicity to upgrade the image of the Traditional doctors. The number of United Clinics in the countryside almost doubled, and the Party now also insisted that Traditional doctors be included in western hospitals and clinic facilities. A major research institute was established in Beijing (China Medical Research Institute) that brought together both kinds of doctors. The China Medical Association, for the first time in 1959, began to include Traditional doctors in its membership (3,000 were enrolled). New hospitals and colleges exclusively for Traditional doctors were established. It was decided to permit older approaches to Traditional medical education through a reinstitution of apprenticeship programs.

Croizier describes the continuing lack of enthusiasm of the western doctors, who dropped out of classes whenever that was possible, ignored the Traditional doctors on staff in the modern hospitals or gave them hopeless cases. In the post-Great Leap period and the 1960s, general public discussion subsided but the practical reality of some forms of integration were firmly in place. Since the experience of the 1950s, the Chinese Communist Party has pushed for an on-going policy of 'combined treatment' of disease. Returning Overseas Chinese Traditional doctors have been welcomed back to the mainland with significant fanfare.

While one of the obstacles to the acceptance of Chung-i has been an inability to explain its theoretical framework in satisfactory scientific terms, Croizier suggests that the following have been the major impetus for the integration: a strong sense of pride that wants to 'creatively inherit' elements of the old national culture, the popularity of the old medicine among the rural masses, the low cost of Traditional treatments in a long period of scarce economic resources and its utilization as a counter-balance to "rectify the undesirable ideological tendencies of the western-trained doctors."

This astute and comprehensive analysis of Chinese health policy with reference to integration provides considerable insight. It can also be seen within the context of an ongoing battle over who would dominate health policy—the conservative bureaucracy at the Ministry of Health or Mao, through the CCP apparatus.

INTEGRATION POLICY EVALUATION: 1949-1976

Lampton sketches out the most comprehensive picture of PRC general health policy evolution, since the Revolution, that is available (Lampton 1977). Included in his larger analysis and history are details of how the integration directive fared during various periods of political and policy changes after 1949. One of Lampton's major theses is that the Ministry of Health was dominated by western-trained physicians who found it difficult to implement Mao's directives because they were seriously incompatible with their own training, orientation and view of how health care could and should be organized and delivered. These are two approaches with significant structural differences and natural built-in conflict.

The twenty-seven years he describes in his book, *The Politics of Medicine in China*, were ones where power and influence alternated between an entrenched bureaucracy that wanted to proceed with administrative prudence and scientific caution, and the CCP moving with a revolutionary fervor to deal with health problems in openly political terms. The direct attention and energy of Party activity emerges to implement a special approach or program; then events weaken that effort and the bureaucracy at the Ministry quietly regains influence and authority. The fluctuating patterns of dominance enhance understanding of Croizier's analysis and etch more deeply the background within which one can understand very current material. Lampton divides the three decades into the following periods as both health policy (normative policy) and implementation (action policy) unfold from Liberation to the Great Leap Forward to the aftermath of the Cultural Revolution.

1949-54 Mao's four principles in health work announced but professional dominance at the Ministry prevails temporarily.

1954-57 Chinese Communist Party pushes for dominance over professionals: Red versus Expert; collectivization pushed.

1958-59 Great Leap Forward: Collectivization intensified including establishment of commune clinics with need to bolster the image of Traditional doctors.

1960–65 Collapse of Great Leap; fragmentation of leadership; power drifts back to Ministry; tight budgets.

1965–69 Cultural Revolution; 23 June 1965 blast at
Ministry; Barefoot Doctor program initiated: study
of Traditional medicine part of training.

1969–77 Aftermath of Cultural Revolution; uncertainty and
confusion.

1973–77 Drift of influence back to Ministry and professionalism.

During the period from 1949–1954, Lampton finds great
resistance on the part of the Ministry of Health to the idea of
union with Traditional doctors and not much active implementation. Actually, it was not until 1954 that the Central
Committee of the Chinese Communist Party moved aggressively on the issue. According to this source, the CCP recognized both the need to utilize all resources in the medical area
where everything was in short supply and also wanted to assert
more control over the medical profession. Mao reasserted the
need to utilize Traditional doctors. During the Great Leap
(1958–1959) rural commune health clinics were promoted along
with further collectivization. These were primarily staffed by
Traditional doctors who were often the only medical personnel
available. Lampton states that several national vice-ministers
who supported extensive use of Traditional doctors obtained
office during this period based on the Traditional medicine
dispute. The Ministry of Health was forced to help bolster the
status of Traditional doctors so that ". . . rural populations
would take treatment in the commune clinics and not flood
urban facilities" (Lampton 1977).

It was during this period that the Ministry did articulate
a detailed policy that tried to encourage the following: (1)
western-trained doctors were to study Traditional medicine; (2)
Traditional doctors were to be placed in western-style facilities;
(3) construction of new Traditional medical schools; and (4)
increased research into Traditional treatment. Lampton
suggests this four-pronged policy had a highly differential fate:
western doctors resisted the additional study of Traditional
medicine and only a relatively small number responded to the
call; where Traditional doctors were given their own departments in western facilities, they fared much better than when

they were assigned to all departments because other physicians 'didn't co-operate much'; in 1957–1958 seventeen new colleges of Traditional medicine were opened with five-year programs.

In 1961, the Bureau of Traditional medicine was shifted out of the Commerce Ministry into the Ministry of Health. A new director was appointed who was a nationally respected Traditional doctor. Lampton describes the new director's position on various issues concerning integration. He wanted to emphasize research and establish more thorough medical education to upgrade Traditional medicine. He preferred a reduction in attempts to integrate with every aspect of western medicine and discouraged western doctors from studying Traditional medicine. He felt this would undercut the ability of Traditional doctors to preserve dominance in their own domain. And he wanted to reduce the popularization of Traditional medicine (e.g., wide-spread teaching of acupuncture) because he felt this 'degraded' the Tradition.

1960 to 1965, the aftermath of the Great Leap agricultural failures, was a period of fragmented leadership and inability of the CCP to sustain its programs. The availability of Traditional herbs dropped with the agricultural problems in the countryside and this affected the ability of Traditional doctors to practice.

From the onset of the Cultural Revolution from 1965 to 1969, the Ministry of Health was under special scrutiny and attack. Mao accused it of neglecting the health needs of the rural population, of being the 'Ministry of Urban Health'. Top officials were replaced with Party cadre who made policy. The Barefoot Doctor program was initiated and became pervasive around the country. Lampton states that there was no clear policy towards Traditional medicine and integration during this period and the time up to Mao's death in 1976. However, he suggests a drift of power back to the old line officials and original policies at the Ministry of Health in the aftermath of the Cultural Revolution. Certain suppositions may therefore be made. Barefoot Doctor training courses and manuals include significant amounts of material from the Tradition. Cultural Revolution fervor would have been directed against western physicians as part of the urban elites Mao attacked during this period. So Traditional doctors' status was probably strengthened and enhanced.

Lampton's final assessment is that in the aftermath of the Cultural Revolution, power gradually drifted back to the Ministry. Earlier professional leaders gradually resumed power reflecting their old emphasis on professionalism and research. However, by this time certain significant changes had already taken place. These included the co-operative medical services of the countryside, the Barefoot Doctor program and the wide dispersal of Traditional doctors throughout the system.

HYPOTHETICAL 'MODES' OF RESPONSE

Mao's original call to integrate the two medical traditions was a general principle, not a pragmatic plan. Mao set policy but did not provide a blueprint for its implementation. That was left to be worked out by the Ministry of Health, Party cadre and individual health facilities. What Croizier and Lampton report suggests that implementation produced a variegated pattern in actual practice. Apparently a variety of plans were attempted, reflecting the changing political situation, shifting definitions of need as well as pragmatic reality. Some plans, once put into effect, fell by the wayside. Others proved more practical and long-lived.

From a sociological point of view, it might be suggested that there were actually four functional modes of response to the policy on integration. These hypothetical modes represent the conceivable ways the policy could be implemented in health care facilities. One, the two medical approaches could be afforded equal status in diagnosis, treatment, medical education. This indeed has been suggested by enthusiastic visitors. Such a mode can be called 'Total Integration' and suggests a combination of parts into a whole (the meaning of integration in common parlance). Two, there could be a division of duties with clearcut responsibilities assigned to each modality: 'Selective Integration'. Third, the path followed could be one of absorption of aspects of Traditional medicine into the practices of western medicine, what could be seen as 'Assimilation' in the sociological sense of accepting a dominant culture and disappearing into it. Fourth, the directive could be ignored, delaying and foot-dragging techniques employed and efforts made to repudiate the policy: 'Rejection'. Thus, assigning Traditional doctors important hospital staff positions with equal status to western physicians would be an example of 'Total Integration'. Deciding that Traditional doctors would treat a pre-determined group of medical problems would be 'Selective Integration'. The CCP post-1950s push for western doctors to utilize both treatment modalities for a treatment of a wide range of illness would be 'Assimilation'. Western doctors dropping out of Traditional courses or giving Traditional doctors impossible cases to treat might be seen as 'Rejection'.

These modalities represent major differences in interpretation of Mao's directive and reflect on the health care system's pragmatic response to the creation of the New Chinese Medicine he called for. They reflect pragmatic responses to the relative importance of Traditional theory, Traditional diagnostic and treatment procedures and Traditional practitioners themselves in the grass roots of the health care system.

What of the current situation, the beginnings of the post-Mao period since 1976 with the Ministry of Health once more dominating health policy evolution? The study tour in August 1979 may provide some clues. It began with a detailed discussion at the China Medical Association where normative policy was described and its problems discussed with considerable frankness (Study Journal 1979).

THE INTEGRATION OF TRADITIONAL AND WESTERN MEDICINE: CURRENT NORMATIVE POLICY?

The China Medical Association whose major purpose is to provide an organization voice for the medical profession, has a variety of tasks. These include internal exchange of medical knowledge, the international exchange of medical information and ideas and the publication of medical journals. It operates under the aegis of the Ministry of Health and acts as a conduit for professional medicines' opinions and positions on a wide variety of pertinent issues. In this capacity, it serves as an advisory arm of the Ministry in the formulation of health policy. Furthermore, it then has responsibility for seeing that the state health policy is promulgated among its members. Its functional relationship to the Ministry is delineated in a comprehensive organizational chart suggested by Lampton, although the role of the CMA has varied considerably over time (Lampton 1980).

A long afternoon briefing with Dr Liu, Vice-President of the China Medical Association in its Beijing headquarters, touched on many aspects of the integration policy and program. A review of Dr Liu's statements and remarks appear to suggest aspects of current normative policy and some of its recent developments and problems.

The Vice-President of the CMA reiterated the four principles of medical and health work which Chairman Mao had proclaimed in 1950.

His statement of the fourth, to combine Traditional doctors with doctors of western medicine, included reference to the fact that this is unique to China. It had a medical tradition with a long history and although western medicine had been introduced about 100 years ago, the country badly needed the two schools because then . . . "the people can create the best medicine for the defense of their health."

It was explained that because of 'limited conditions' and the oppression of the Kuomintang, Chung-i experienced slow development in theory, in diagnostic approaches and in treatment procedures over the period of its long history. This was so particularly because it was not able to absorb the modern knowledge of western medicine. Traditional medicine ". . . is still incomplete and . . . modern knowledge (will be used) to make it clear and to bring it up to date."

Training of medical manpower was the first issue he covered. In general, Traditional medicine composes 30 percent of the curricula in the various levels of western medical schools. In the special colleges of Traditional medicine, 30 percent of study is in western techniques. Pilot studies are currently being conducted to see how best to teach both. Some 10,000 western physicians now have additional training in the Traditional which usually takes two years of in-service work. They are considered the backbone of current medical education and research in Chung-i. But Dr Liu expressed some disappointment in how small this number is. The key to the success of integration, Dr Liu asserted, is acceptance by the western-trained doctors and "it is difficult for them." He also emphasized that there are not very many really well-experienced doctors of Traditional medicine in the whole country at this time.

He spoke about the great wealth of herbs grown in China, particularly in the South and how this is a significant contribution to the low medical fees in the country. The economic advantages of Traditional medicine are considered of great importance. The question of how widely Traditional medicine is accepted among the urban and rural population was raised. The general assessment was that since city populations had been more exposed to western medicine, they were more widely accepting of it particularly since Traditional medicine, he said, "wasn't developed before." It is in the countryside that the greatest utilization and acceptance of Traditional medicine and practitioners can be found.

Dr Liu often used anecdotal material to describe the success of particular Traditional treatment approaches. Traditional fracture treatment which combines mobilization and demobilization has reduced healing time in selected cases—one-third the time necessary with strictly western approaches. As far as acupuncture is concerned, a skilled doctor can treat sixty to seventy varieties of the "common and recurring" diseases with success and these include "many that western medicine can't deal with." Dr Liu included a story about his own personal success treating then Vice-Chairman Deng for a case of arthritis . . . "I treated him with acupuncture and it took one month to cure it." When asked whether his contention that Traditional medicine is useful for some sixty to seventy varieties of disease is based on systematic research and controlled studies, his response was that he is referring primarily to the past thirty years of clinical practice and some controlled studies. One controlled study divided patients with tonsillitis into two groups, one treated with penicillin and the other with acupuncture treatment. The results, he said, "were the same." He reiterated that disbelief was often widespread among western-trained physicians but after personally practicing Traditional medicine, he made the generalization that they are convinced that it actually works and even achieves better results in some cases.

Research on herbal medicines and on the mechanisms of acupuncture are currently carried out at various medical universities and academies by both western and Traditional doctors although it was not clear whether they work together or in separate laboratories.

Perhaps one of the most revealing exchanges occurred when Dr Liu was asked if Traditional doctors belong to the China Medical Association. He answered that the Traditional doctors had their own association—the All China Association of Traditional Chinese Medicine which was formed after a very recent (May 1979) conference.

What was the purpose of establishing a separate organization, was the next question, if the goal is to unify the two approaches?

The response was that the two schools do not "speak the same languages and that the research interests are not the same."

The discussion concluded with a number of observations. Dr Liu pointed out that the interest in Traditional medicine has spread to many countries, some of whom are conducting their own research as the Japanese are doing with acupuncture. Many students and physicians from the Third World countries are coming to study Traditional therapies in China. But much work remains to be done in improving and developing Traditional medicine.

Dr Liu said he hoped medical workers in the USA and PRC could learn from each other. Perhaps, he remarked, China could import American technology and export Traditional medicine (Study Journal 1979).

Commentary

The CMA visit provided the opportunity to hear a rendition of current policy concerning the integration and to begin an assessment of its realities as well. Many of the themes established in the Croizier and Lampton material are found reflected in this recent CMA discussion. One can see both a continued commitment to integration as well as the problems that were present at the initiation of the policy.

Despite thirty years of effort, Dr Liu's remarks are strewn with hints about the difficulties and doubts that not only remain but in some instances, may have grown stronger. The path to a 'United Front' of the two medicines appears to have been neither smooth nor enthusiastically travelled. Mao chiefly indicated that the integration was to come about in terms of a map drawn in western bio-medical style, hence it was the western doctors who were to guide the venture. But three decades later, "it is (still) difficult for western doctors to accept." The 10,000 who have now studied both styles are not considered enough. Problems of communication between the two groups persist and apparently, Traditional doctors are no longer accepted for membership in the CMA as was the policy in the late 1950s. And the new organization for Traditional doctors is a brand new creation. It appears, then, that there has been a very recent decision made that is a clear comment on the continuing differences between the two groups. Whether this is the outcome of decisions by western doctors that Traditionals cannot function appropriately in the western-style professional organization or whether Traditional doctors have acted out of a desire for autonomy as a base for strengthening their status is not known. However, there is here substantial evidence of the continuing doubts and resistance that thirty years of experience have not softened or lessened.

Much in the briefing also pointed to a strong need for research in a number of areas. Despite the fact that research institutes have been established since the mid-1950s and scientific study is taking place in many medical schools, it is clinical evidence and personal experience with Traditional treatment that are cited as the basis for utilization of Traditional methods. Convincing evidence is stronger in some areas than in others. For example, Traditional approaches to fractures seem well established as do treatments for acute abdomines. Controlled, double-blind studies were not mentioned but rather simple comparisons between two groups of patients where no information is available about how they were chosen and how the experimental comparison was conducted. Several times Dr Liu reiterated that not enough research had been carried out.

Research in a different topic was mentioned as well. Pilot studies on how to teach the two medicines together have recently been instituted. This suggests on-going concern with educational effectiveness in both western and Traditional schools.

Other problems remain such as a continuing reluctance among the urban population to accept Traditional medicine, a dearth of "very many really well-trained Traditional doctors" across the country, and a continuing need to bring Traditional medicine up to date. Dr Liu's historical recollections have conveniently ignored the early Communist criticisms concerning the inadequacies of Chung-i, imputing them instead only to the Kuomintang.

Yet a commitment to integration was firmly and repeatedly stated throughout the briefing. Dr Liu said, "We badly need both schools (of medicine)." He enumerated many conditions that respond to Traditional treatment, mentioning individual cases where it worked, while also pointing out its economic advantages. He was proud of the fact that this aspect of the PRC system has received world-wide attention. And he reflected a continuing commitment to pursuing the integration policy.

We left the CMA briefing with a number of clear messages, the primary one being that although western-trained doctors remain to be convinced and many original objections and questions persist, practical integration is a reality. Dr Liu ended the briefing by saying that with the new commitment to modernization, they have a great interest in obtaining modern medical technology yet he also made it clear that the inclusion of Traditional medicine would go on as well. The commitment to integration continues strong, albeit shot through with contradiction and ambivalence.

It was fortunate that the CMA briefing took place the first day of the study tour. With this as an introduction to possible current normative policy, it was then possible to view subsequent health facility visits as examples of that policy in action. While not approximating any sort of systematic research, a great deal of information on integration was gathered that reflect patterns of integration as well as perceptual attitudes about the uses of Traditional medicine. A review of this material will permit not only a comparison of action policy with normative policy as described by the CMA, but some insights into which of the four modes of integration can be found and under what circumstances.

EXAMPLES OF INTEGRATION: OBSERVATIONS AND INFORMATION COLLECTED IN 1979

The study tour's August 1979 material can be grouped and categorized in a number of distinct ways. It includes the following: (1) personal statements on preference for Traditional or western medicine; (2) examples of institutional approaches to integration; (3) a list of conditions being treated with Traditional and/or combined approaches; and (4) descriptions of approaches to teaching the Tradition in a variety of medical schools and settings.

Personal statements

On some two dozen occasions, it was possible to ask people directly whether they preferred western or Traditional medicine and gather responses from men and women, young and old in the variety of places we visited. While this can, by no stretch, be called a survey or be considered representative, the responses are revealing. The modal group did not use Traditional medicine at all. Well under half claim to utilize both kinds of medications and these were evenly divided between the sexes and age groupings. A very small number claim to use only Traditional medicine. Among all those engaged in conversation, however there was common agreement that Traditional Chinese medicine (i.e., herbs, acupuncture, and herbal mixtures) was useful for 'common' illnesses like colds, simple abdominal problems like stomach aches, headaches, chronic conditions and prevention. It was widely stated that Traditional medicine had fewer side effects.

Obversely, western medicine is seen as best for serious illness like hypertension and problems requiring surgery. The common remark was that "western medicine works more quickly." However, even in this small sample of personal statements, there were conflicting perceptions and experiences. Different people claimed opposite choices for treatment of headaches, appendicitis, fever and bad colds. Differences of opinion apparently exist in the same family as well. A mother of three grown children in the Beijing Moon Temple Gate neighborhood remarked that while one daughter prefers

Traditional medicine, the other chooses western because "herbs are very bitter." Her son, on the other hand, takes western medicines because "it works more quickly than herbs" and that is her own preference as well.

Another example of mixed choices is reflected in a conversation with a sophisticated Beijing urbanite who discussed varying choices for herself, her husband and her infant son. For the infant, a western medical approach is preferred and her husband makes this choice for himself as well. For her own back problem she takes Traditional treatment, uses both for a cough but in a case of serious illness, western medicine "is best because it is quicker."

In several instances, informants observed that western medicine was more popular in the cities and among the young. Yet a contradiction to this came in a statement made by the Director of the Home for the Respected Elderly outside of Fushen. He stated, in response to a direct question, that the residents of the facility use acupuncture but prefer western medicine because they get quicker results. And that they keep western medicine in their rooms such as pain killers and hypertensives.

One of the strongest personal statements made in support of Traditional medicine was from a young man of twenty-nine who came from a rural peasant background. He is now living in a large metropolitan area and has received training as a teacher. He is employed in a factory 'after hours college' where he teaches English. This man expressed fervent loyalty to Chairman Mao and spoke of how the revolution had changed his life, providing opportunities unthought of by his rural parents. He also stated that the Chinese people are particularly attached to Traditional medicine since it is part of their national heritage. Adding an aside, he thought it might be necessary to use western medicine for very serious illness.

In the same metropolitan area, an interview with an urban-bred young woman of about the same age, who had been brought up by well-educated parents, revealed a different point of view. She stated firmly that young people much prefer western medicine, as did she. Going on to soften this declaration somewhat, she said that sometimes she did use Traditional medicine for colds and that on one occasion she went to see a

Traditional doctor. She said she found it surprising that he was able to diagnose without asking any questions.

Comparing this minute, grab sample of peoples opinions and preferences with how our host at the China Medical Association described preferences in general among the population, rather remarkable agreement is found. Greatest doubts exist among urbanites, with under half of these twenty-four informants using both kinds of medicine and emphasizing Traditional for minor illness and western for the more serious. They agree that there are fewer side effects with herbs but that quicker results are obtained with western. The contradictory claims of usefulness for specific illnesses reflect the CMA statement that much research is needed to establish the clear cut efficacy of various herbs and traditional treatments. Utilization seems in many instances arbitrary and individualized.

This small sample suggests that individuals are practicing 'Selective' integration with urbanites making a variety of choices and utilizing Traditional medicine for more minor ailments. The most whole-hearted enthusiasm for Traditional medicine was expressed by the individual with the most rural background although even here, there is recognition that western is necessary for more serious illness. There is the suggestion that in the minds of some elderly citizens, who knew the old society well, that western medicine is preferable.

This is an area for systematic research but indications are that some people, while using Traditional medicine, chose carefully and are ready to turn to modern approaches for serious problems. The continued skepticism in the cities that the CMA mentioned was reflected in this small sample of the population.

Approaches to Integration in Health Facilities

Despite the short period of time actually spent in the People's Republic of China, the study group managed to visit small health clinics in factories, a neighborhood lane and a commune, three western style urban teaching hospitals two of which were advanced specialty and research hospitals, a college of Traditional medicine and attached hospital; a home for the elderly, a rural commune district hospital; a county hospital and nurses' school, a workers' convalescent home, an urban street pharmacy and a municipal health bureau.

In these various contexts it was possible to observe some patterns of how Traditional medicine is structured within facilities and hence obtain clues about organizational responses to integration (Study Journal 1979).

Every facility visited is utilizing some forms of Traditional treatment. Sometimes the same disease or illness entity is being treated differently (in one place with herbs; in another with acupuncture) but in each health unit from neighborhood lane health station to Harbin Teaching Hospital #2 where liver transplant experiments are taking place, mention was made of utilizing the Traditional methods. Separate outpatient departments of Traditional medicine existed in all of the hospitals and clinics visited. In-patient departments were found in one of the western-style hospitals but not at the other two, although in-patient departments were in place at the three rural hospitals. The logic of how the departments of Traditional medicine are being utilized is not altogether clear.

On an in-patient basis, they appear to be equated with internal medicine and surgery and on an out-patient basis, with general medical clinics. There is a great deal of inconsistency here since many of the same conditions are being treated in a department of internal medicine and a department of Traditional medicine. The same might be said of surgery and Traditional medicine, particularly with reference to 'acute abdomines' such as appendicitis, pancreatitis and gall bladder disease cases of which are to be found in all three departments. Apparently, this is not essentially a matter of patient preference. In these instances we were told that a patient might choose to present himself at a Traditional medicine outpatient clinic but once diagnosed, the doctors would have the final say as to the treatment procedures and the in-patient department assignment. More serious cases are treated with western techniques but no consistent policy exists for cases in the 'gray' areas between mild and serious.

Scrutinizing more closely the one Traditional in-patient department which was visited in the Shenyang China Medical University, its department head is of particular interest. She was originally trained as a western physician at CMU, practiced for some nine years and then responded to Chairman Mao's call for western doctors to study and become Traditional physicians as well. Her Traditional training was for one year. She is one of the 10,000 who is technically qualified to practice both. She stated that an integrated approach to treatment is practiced within her department although she tries to emphasize Traditional medicine.

The one other mention of an in-patient Traditional medicine department was at the Tong Ren Municipal General Hospital in Beijing. Here the situation was dramatically different. This hospital is an important tertiary care facility that specializes in ophthalmology and ENT and has two research institutes attached. In these areas it receives patients from all over the country. It also operates as an emergency center for all of Beijing and functions as a referral center for local hospitals in a wide variety of illness categories. It has a number of out-patient clinics that see 3,200 people a day and actually services a population of one million people. It was the most sophisticated of the facilities visited with 380 doctors, 350 nurses, 180 technicians and 150 medical students receiving clinical training as well as nursing students. A tour included the medical and surgical wards and an out-patient Traditional medicine room.

In this out-patient department which has been in the hospital since 1954, patients were being treated for post-partum problems, spasms of facial nerves, hypertension and bursitis. Apparently there had been no in-patient Traditional beds although the out-patient department had been in place for twenty-five years. In response to a question about the future of Traditional medicine in the Tong Ren hospital, the director said,

> We have been asked to establish a new ward for the Traditional medicine department . . . we've been required to give thirty beds . . . but haven't done so yet, so we give the patients combined treatment and put them in the internal medicine or surgery department.

Another subject was raised at Tong Ren, the question of what patients they referred to the Traditional hospital in Beijing. When asked for several recent examples of the cases, they

mentioned referral of patients with aplastic anemia and throm-
bocytopenia. Could this be an example of dumping difficult
patients?

The distant rural countryside hospitals have both in- and
out-patient Traditional departments as well as additional units
reflecting closer commitment to integration. For example, the
county hospital and the commune district hospital have extensive herbal gardens (the county growing 180 different herbs
and the commune over 300 species). Both of these medicinal
gardens were tended by elderly Traditional doctors or
herbalists. Both locations also have facilities for drying and
storing herbs and making their own pills and other medications.

Two other facilities merit special description: a convalescent hospital and a Traditional college and hospital. The
Harbin Workers Convalescent Home is located on an island in
the Songhua River, and surrounded by a formal garden equal
to its English models, has no specific department of Traditional
medicine but Traditional modalities are utilized extensively
throughout and join both medical traditions in unique ways
that will be discussed further on. Many Traditional doctors are
on its staff.

At the Shenyang College of Traditional Medicine,
integration proceeds within a distinctly different frame of
reference. It appeared to be more full-blown integration, closer
to equal status. Western bio-medical science is afforded a place
of respect along side of Traditional theory. It will be important
to see, over time, if it displaces the Traditional theory
completely. The afternoon visit however, did not permit
examination of all pertinent subjects and issues. This Institute
includes both a Traditional hospital and medical school founded
in 1958 but based on a former Traditional school and hospital.
It currently has 400 in-patient beds, 1,500 students and 1,800
teachers and medical workers.

The hospital director who served as one of our hosts was
a western trained physician who later also took training in
Traditional medicine. His introductory remarks included an
historical analysis stating that past . . .

reactionary governments had moved to eliminate
Traditional medicine ever since western medicine had

come to China . . . but Liberation and Mao had given Chung-i new life . . . ever since, there has been great development.

It was particularly interesting to hear him describe the four major functions of the hospital which were to (1) treat common diseases in combined theory, (2) provide clinical experiences for students, (3) conduct research in Traditional medicine, and (4) train western doctors in Traditional medicine. Even more revealing was a recital of this Traditional hospital's department structure: internal medicine, surgery, ENT, obstetrics-gynecology, pediatrics and radiology. Surgery and radiology, of course, were never part of Traditional medicine and signifies a very modern addition.

We also visited an acupuncture out-patient clinic and witnessed demonstrations of tooth extraction with acupressure, cauterization of tonsils, acupuncture treatment with moxibustion for stroke victims and cupping with heated bamboo sections for bursitis.

An impressive and well-kept specimen room displayed some 1,200 medicinal products from plants and animals. The Institute is carrying out research on both the theoretical and clinical aspects of Traditional medicine. They "emphasize (research into) what kinds of disease can be treated effectively with herbs and on the principal channels in acupuncture." Researchers are 'very, very experienced' Traditional doctors, newly-trained graduates and a small number of western physicians with additional training in the Tradition.

The education program of the students, along with Traditional subjects includes physiological anatomy, pharmacological chemistry, X-ray diagnosis and 'part' of western diagnosis. Furthermore, the statement was made that applicants to this school are expected to pass the same national entrance examination now required of all medical school applicants. According to reports this emphasizes chemistry, math, physics and foreign language requiring a senior middle school education.

The director of the Acupuncture Department discussed the current state and future of Traditional medicine. "So far we have realized that the integration is better than treatment with Traditional medicine alone." He cited several examples:

"with gall stones X-ray provides information as to where the stone is and whether it has been passed; in shoulder para-arthritis the use of Traditional massage, while effective, can cause sharp pain so western pain-killers are useful." He also enumerated the benefits of acupuncture anesthesia: "the patient is conscious and can cooperate, there is less bleeding, no side effects and faster recovery." A seventy-year-old Traditional doctor who had studied with a nineteenth century Master described a puzzling case that repeated efforts by western doctors had failed to cure while Traditional medicine was highly effective.

When asked why there was not now an integration of professional organizations, the response was that "there are still too many problems to be solved and not enough doctors know both medicines equally well. If a western doctor can practice Traditional Chinese medicine as well as he does western medicine, then the integration of both will come about." But both the acupuncturist and the older Traditional doctor were optimistic about the integration. The Chinese people, young and old, they both claimed, prefer their Chung-i and therefore it has a "bright future."

The future was articulated in quite another fashion by the Traditional hospital director who was asked about future acquisitions for the hospital. A hypothetical question was posed: if the State gave you 100,000 Yuan more next year for your budget, what would you want to get? His answer was swift and short: "a CAT scanner." This, of course, is one of the most sophisticated pieces of diagnostic technology available in western medicine.

In all the other facilities visited, doctors of Traditional medicine are on staff working in out-patient settings that specialize in Traditional techniques, the most common of which are acupuncture, moxibustion and cupping. The Traditional hospital demonstrated acupressure tooth extraction but a factory hospital dental clinic said that was not in practice in their facility.

Across the patchwork quilt of approaches to the integration that emerged during the trip, one repeated motif was apparent: that the utilization of Traditional medicine was economical. From the most advanced tertiary care hospital in Beijing to the distant rural commune district hospital in KaiAn the statement was the same. It is always cheaper to use acupuncture and herbs. The director of Tong Ren Hospital, a sophisticated medical researcher at Harbin #2 Hospital, the vice-president of China Medical University, the director of the county hospital in Nong-An, the director of the commune hospital all emphasized the importance of Traditional treatments to their budgets. Some of the figures are worth noting.

At Harbin Teaching Hospital, #2, treatment of appendicitis with herbs costs twenty Yuan while surgery costs forty to fifty Yuan (1979 exchange rate one Yuan = $1.68). At Nong An County Hospital an appendicitis treated traditionally costs five Yuan while surgery is thirty Yuan. These figures seem to reflect differences between a large metropolitan area and a rural town as well as the fact that Nong An had its own herb garden. Both are examples, however, of the savings accrued through the use of Traditional treatment. The rural facilities reported this with what seemed like pride. The urban statements seemed more in the context of a defense.

Are there hints that may be garnered from this anecdotal material as to the more general patterns of institutional integration?

Generalizations about this limited material suggest that western biomedical frames of reference very much prevail. Outside of acupuncturists who were directors of acupuncture treatment clinics, all encounters with directors of Traditional medicine in-patient facilities indicated they were first western-trained doctors with some additional minimal training in the Tradition. This is particularly noteworthy at the Traditional hospital itself. Are Traditional doctors with final powers of decision-making in charge at any in-patient settings? The rural facilities, particularly in the more distant countryside exhibit more enthusiasm for the integration and may permit more autonomy to practitioners but also are more obviously dependent on the economy utilization of herbal medicines permits in their budgets. One urban hospital in Beijing has been able to resist establishing a separate in-patient ward for almost thirty years.

Nowhere were there examples of Traditional doctors having the authority to utilize western treatment procedures although information from other sources suggest that Traditional doctors with some western training are prescribing

60

antibiotics. Everywhere western-trained physicians combined both techniques for their patients. Finally, a western bio-medical science frame of reference for disease diagnosis and treatment prevailed at each facility visited. Even the Traditional practitioners are in the throes of embracing it as a look at the list of the Traditional hospital's departments and their medical school program reveals.

Kleinman Observations

Our material can be compared with observations reported by Kleinman based on a rural health tour taken in 1978 (Kleinman 1978). Kleinman, a physician and anthropologist who speaks Chinese, has written extensively on Traditional Chinese medicine and is perhaps better able to assess the nature of the integration than any other recent visitor. He concluded that utilization of Chung-i is taking place almost exclusively within the framework of western medical science and theory. He describes how western medical concepts guide the empirical use of Traditional treatment procedures. Traditional diagnostic concepts are usually translated into western medical idioms and when Traditional medical terminology is utilized, it is not in the original Traditional sense but as a translation of western medical beliefs. He also mentions the isolation of Traditional doctors in separate departments.

One of the most interesting conversations he reports is with a physician who was Deputy Director of the Hsing Hui County Hospital of Traditional Chinese Medicine. Kleinman asked the director to respond to his impressions that "western medical ideas (guided) the empirical use of Chinese medicines and (that) Traditional Chinese medical concepts (were being) translated in western medical idiom." The director responded affirmatively and said that was indeed happening and it represented progress. He is quoted as saying:

What is important is effective treatment. Even in the past, the ideas changed. But now we have the oppor-tunity to understand what we do scientifically and to use what is effective from both systems . . .

The 1979 study tour material reveals similar patterns and statements. However, many more instances of western doctors utilizing mixed modalities were indicated in 1979 than what Kleinman reports from his information.

Is this integration or is it western medicine assimilating selected treatment modalities and Traditional medicine grasping for a future by enmeshing itself in a structure of western medical explanation? The overall pattern is a combination of Selective and Assimilative integration with western doctors doing the 'assimilating'. The only institution approaching 'Total Integration' was the Traditional hospital and medical school.

Examples of Assimilative Integration in Treatment

Over the span of the study tour some forty different conditions were mentioned as being treated with Traditional techniques (almost always herbs and/or acupuncture) or with combined treatment (Study Journal 1979). These ranged from simple colds and sore throats to acute abdomines such as pancreatis and gall stones to cerebral embolism and cardiovascular disease. A complete list of all conditions mentioned as well as cases presented to the study group can be found in the Study Journal. It is difficult to make even superficial generalizations about this list since information is incomplete. The problems mentioned are a conglomeration of highly disparate situations where questions of direct and indirect effects of various medications would have to be addressed as well as issues having to do with self-limiting illness and natural remission. Presumably, the Chinese are currently conducting research to sort out these issues and establish objective evidence.

The overall approach however, seems to be combining western drugs and other treatment modalities with herbal prescriptions and acupuncture both at the same time or differentially throughout the course of illness. For specific examples, the reader is referred to the Study Journal. Here the extensive list is divided into Simple Diseases, Chronic Illness, Acute Abdomines and a disparate grouping: Other.

The wide-ranging quality of this list, which was gathered in a sixteen-day period of time, reflects some of the same diversity found among the personal statements. It should be noted that many of the serious illnesses were mentioned in the more rural settings where there may be greater shortages of western drugs, technology and western-trained personnel. It is also possible that the diagnoses themselves are less reliable in rural areas (Lampton 1980). One overall assessment, however, is that the range of the list reflects lack of scientific validation and conclusive evidence, broad clinical experimentation and different clinical experience. How much shortages are a factor cannot be ascertained. What is clear is extensive mixed use by western doctors. For whichever reasons, and these no doubt include clinical efficacy, western doctors are assimilating Traditional practices.

Another order of integration can be seen in the innovative joining of science and Traditional medicine on a technological level. Examples of this were seen in many locations but the fullest panoply in one health facility was at the Harbin Workers Convalescent Home which specialized in the treatment of chronic diseases. Here one can witness the electrical heating of glass globes for cupping treatment, the electrical heating of herb packets which were seen placed on legs for the treatment of chronic pain, heads for chronic headaches and chests for patients with heart problems. It was not possible to ascertain how effective these techniques were.

Electrical twirling of acupuncture needles was demonstrated as well as a unique technique that was not witnessed elsewhere. This involved the use of a weak laser light beamed at an acupuncture point in the throat of a patient suffering from chronic bronchitis. The idea seemed to be that the light would penetrate the point just as an acupuncture needle and moxibustion (the burning of a herb over an acupuncture point) do. This treatment was described as experimental but is a vivid example of the 'technical' level of integration that is also going on. Electrical twirling of acupuncture needles is found everywhere. Laser lights on acupuncture points is a recent experiment indicating a commitment to continuing the search for how treatments can be combined.

The Teaching of Traditional Medicine in Various Settings

Every teaching facility visited engaged in teaching students at least some aspects of Traditional medicine although only general information was obtainable (Study Journal 1979). At the China Medical University in Shenyang, it was pointed out that foreign students attend the University in a steady stream, particularly to study the Traditional techniques like acupuncture. Chinese students of course rotate through the in-patient Traditional Medicine Department as part of their overall clinical training. Training also takes place in the out-patient room for electrical acupunture therapy. It was impossible to ascertain, from brief observation, how highly the staff regards the Traditional techniques and what attitudes they convey to students. Research in the USA indicates that faculty attitudes are an important influence on students. This would be an important area for research in the PRC.

Harbin Medical Institute #2 Hospital is part of a large medical complex that includes a medical university and a sophisticated research center. It was mentioned that a current item of study was the mechanisms of acupuncture as an anesthesia. It was clear from all the cases presented to the study group that selected herbal and acupunture treatments were widely used by the western-trained physicians in the hospital. There were Traditional practitioners on the staff but one got the impression that they played minor roles. There were no direct indications that Traditional medicine is widely taught in this setting other than what clinical students would see in the forms of combined treatments utilized in the wards.

There was also an opportunity to obtain information about the teaching of Traditional medicine at TsingTao Medical College from a professor of pharmacology on the faculty who spoke to the group privately. A department of Traditional medicine exists in the college and some 300 out of 2,000 enrolled at the school study in this department every year. The modern textbooks used at TsingTao contain material on "selected Traditional medicines which have been scientifically analyzed." More research is going on at the college to analyze, verify and prove the advantages of certain herbal medicines. It was clear, however, that the teaching and research activities of the Department of Traditional Medicine and the Department of Pharmacology were both overlapping yet distinctly separate.

The Learning Institute of Traditional Medicine in Harbin has already been discussed. Here, of course, Traditional medicine is dominant in the curriculum but with a strong infusion of western studies such as anatomy, X-ray diagnostics, pharmacological chemistry, and other western diagnostic techniques. One got the impression that the Traditional and western departments were quite separate domains. For example, the herbal display room, a large well-kept and impressive facility with examples of some 1,200 plant and animal specimens teaches students where the specimens are found and which part is medicinally useful. Pharmacological chemistry is a completely separate enterprise although a well-integrated education program might have combined them for teaching purposes.

One additional teaching program was described at facilities in more remote, rural areas. Nong An County Hospital has a School of Nursing as well as a Barefoot Doctors training program. Its Department of Traditional Medicine appears to have extensive support. One of the first statements in a briefing by the hospital's director was that they "take very seriously" their work in integrating western and Traditional medicine and that "special study" programs have been instituted for this purpose. Furthermore, all staff and students assist in maintaining their one hectare herb garden. This facility claimed use of herbs and acupuncture in combined treatment of disease in the most extensive list of conditions described anywhere. So nursing and Barefoot Doctor students would get more clinical exposure than students in other western-style hospitals, clinics and medical schools.

Superficial material indicates, then, that Traditional treatment techniques are taught everywhere but usually through separate departments. The more urban facilities and the most sophisticated maintain the most separation and do the least teaching. The rural setting evinces the most extensive teaching program. However, everywhere normative policy is described as being in effect. This is an area where detailed research will be needed to reveal the extent to which Traditional medicine is taught, what specifically is taught, and how enthusiastically it is taught.

Nothing in any of the material collected provides any clues as to why the 'pilot studies' in integrated teaching mentioned at the CMA are needed or what form they may be taking. It may be assumed that teaching approaches were left to the individual units, that the results have not been satisfactory and that there is now a desire for more uniform and productive approaches.

NORMATIVE POLICY AND ACTION POLICY: AN OVERVIEW

China Medical Association officials described normative policy on the integration of Traditional and western medicine in a highly dichotomous fashion. While beginning and ending with a firm, clear acceptance of Mao Tse-tung's early enunciation of this basic principle to guide health workers in the New China, the briefing also reflected continued skepticism. While emphasizing that Traditional medicine was economical and found clinically useful for a variety of common and chronic illnesses, the research to date apparently has not convinced western-trained physicians to embrace the integration wholeheartedly. Traditional and western physicians remain separated professionally after thirty years, and still do not share a common idiom. The 10,000 western doctors who have studied Traditional medicine are not enough yet to bridge the gap between the two worlds of medicine. And it is western medicine that has to be convinced in order for the new Chinese Medicine that Mao hoped to be created. Normative policy then, was projected as a mixture of commitment and question, reflecting the continued dominance of a western frame of reference.

A summary of the study material corroborates that a great deal, but not all, of normative policy is reflected as action policy. Recalling the earlier discussion of what forms integration might take in practice, a review of the personal statements, functional relationships in institutions, clinical examples and approaches to teaching provide the following pattern of actual integration.

Personal interest in and stated utilization of medicine and practitioners reflects *selective* integration on the part of less than half the consumers of health care who were interviewed. That is, among those who use both modalities, a clear division of application emerges. Young, old, male, female reflect almost unanimous agreement that western treatment should be sought for serious illness and that Traditional approaches are useful for 'common' illness and prevention. Many city people, however, do not use Traditional medicine at all. Statements of skepticism and rejection were expressed by urban citizens while greatest enthusiasm came from rural settings.

The one noteworthy contradiction is the information from the Home for the Respected Elderly. Here a combination of age and chronic illness should have Traditional medicine more highly regarded and broadly utilized. Can one speculate that in keeping with a commitment to provide these elderly with 'the best', western treatment is emphasized? Thirty years of integration, and Traditional medicine has not been fully embraced.

Functioning institutional and clinical integration, with one notable exception, can most accurately be described as *Selective* and *Assimilative*. Separate departments exist throughout the system suggesting a division of duties with Traditional doctors treating common and chronic illness. However, western practitioners widely utilize Traditional treatments along with the western in an approach that assimilates herbal remedies and acupuncture to western theory, diagnosis and treatment just as the recent (1954) discovery of the analgesic effects of acupuncture have been *Selectively* utilized in certain surgical procedures.

Complete division of duties, however, does not exist. Blurring of cases is found everywhere with similar problems being treated in out-patient clinics and in-patient medical/surgery wards and in-patient Traditional medicine wards.

Traditional medicine and practitioners are found everywhere but dominated by a western medical science frame of reference and dominated by western-trained physicians. From the Tong-Ren Hospital in Beijing where there is still successful resistance to establishing Traditional in-patient beds, to the China Medical University where the director of the Traditional In-Patient Ward is originally trained in the western style, to Nong An County where 50 percent of the Barefoot Doctors were formerly Traditional doctors (seeking stable legitimization by changing their health worker designation?), institutional arrangements leave the western doctors in control, utilizing combined treatment extensively but on their own terms. And everywhere explaining this as economically desirable as well as clinically efficacious.

There is however, one excellent example of *Total* integration and equal status for both medicines: The Traditional College and Hospital. Here, it is declared, combining western medicine improves care. Here western diagnostic approaches are both taught and utilized. A surgery department has been instituted and here Traditional theory, diagnosis and treatment are in high esteem, studied, researched and utilized throughout. Yet even here, the director of the hospital was first trained as a western-style doctor.

Much of normative policy reflecting the continued skepticism of the western doctors and their continued dominance in practice consistently appeared in all facilities visited.

Ranging over the extensive list of disease, illness and health problems mentioned throughout, one finds simple or common illness, chronic problems and a wide-ranging list of others some of which would have to be classed as serious. The picture is a confusing one. It is more complex than the normative policy that suggested a division of labor between common and serious health problems. A great deal more information would be needed on a case-by-case basis. Where this is available, it is clear Traditional herbs and acupuncture have been *Assimilated* and combined with western treatment. In the convalescent home this was more extensive than anywhere else, reflecting the normative claims for Traditional medicine's usefulness in chronic illness.

The possibilities for research are great, posing difficult questions of proven efficacy, self-limiting and placebo effects and natural remission. However, western medicine addresses similar questions often without being certain of how to design reliable, controlled studies.

Normative policy does not actually capture the practice realities here. Traditional approaches are used much more broadly than just for simple and chronic illness as the CMA briefing claimed. Perhaps this reflects individual clinical experience, lack of persuasive research and lack of western medicines and equipment, particularly in the countryside.

Most likely, it reflects the paucity of concrete and widely influential research with definitive results.

Opinions on advantages and disadvantages of Traditional medicine reflect agreement everywhere with statements made at the CMA. However, no one raised two interesting points made at the CMA: that some herbs are too expensive and that there are not enough "well-experienced doctors of Traditional medicine" in the country. What these statements might hint at is not clear.

The fourth possible reaction to the call for integration, *Rejection* was observed in one hospital that has resisted an in-patient Traditional department for years. There are also innuendoes that Traditional theory is not of interest to non-Traditional practitioners. Research is being conducted on western scientific terms so that it is hypothesized that acupuncture changes bio-medical actions of the body or has neurophysiological impact, and that herbs have a natural, chemically potent ingredient that can be isolated and identified. Traditional theory itself is not used as an explanatory model.

The realities of integration may be systematically diagrammed in Figure 2.1.

No western-trained doctor expressed interest in Traditional medicine theory. The interest was in establishing the scientific basis of selected Traditional treatment practices. There were examples of Traditional doctors using western diagnostic techniques but no examples of the obverse. Research appears to proceed utilizing scientific criteria although 'clinical experience' was the favorite reference for establishing efficacy of Traditional treatments. Traditional doctors presumably continue to use Traditional diagnosis but are moving to strengthen it with western diagnostic approaches. western medicine clearly dominates and controls the character of the mandated integration. And what it has mandated to date is the *Assimilation* of selected treatment modalities for selected illnesses and the control of Traditional practitioners in health facilities either through isolation or putting previously trained western doctors in charge. Further, there is *Selection* taking place in assigning Traditional medicine a role in primary care, chronic illness, pain management and other areas. By hypothesizing four modes of integration, one is able to get

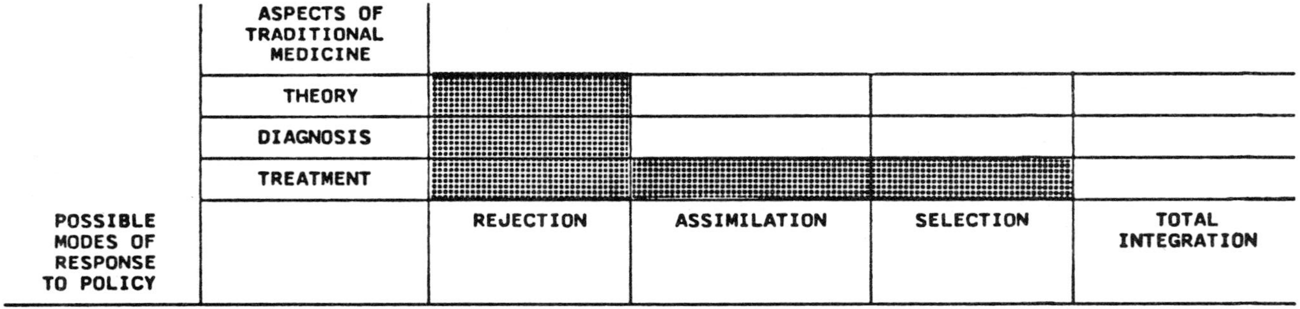

Figure 2.1
Actual Response to Integration Policy

below the surface, look at the implementation of normative policy and see what is happening in actual, practice settings.

The larger action picture, quite closely reflective of normative policy which gets beyond the simple, surface acceptance of the directive to integrate, reveals active and extensive *Assimilation* and *Selection* of certain traditional treatment modalities and *Rejection* of theory and diagnosis. Only in a Traditional setting did we see any signs of *Total* integration.

Chairman Mao would not have been altogether unhappy with the results of that political directive to the People's Republic of China health workers at their First National Conference in 1950. He laid out the principle and left the pragmatics to be worked out. But he wanted Chung-i to be brought into the modern world, to be made scientific. It has indeed experienced an impressive revitalization in contemporary times, being utilized by men and women of science who continue to search for its scientific basis. However, the 'United Front' Mao called for has not materialized.

CONCLUDING ANALYSIS

It is clear that from the beginning, the western-trained physicians resisted Chairman Mao's insistence that Traditional doctors and practices be integrated into the health care system. A variety of strategies were utilized by the Party to accomplish their end, and these strategies varied, depending on other programs the Party was pushing. So, during the Great Leap Forward when rural health clinics were established as part of the agricultural collectivization process, Traditional doctors were almost the only practitioners available to staff them. Their status had to be enhanced. At the same time, the Party sought to assert its dominance over western physicians as part of its Red versus Expert drive.

Building more Traditional medical schools, training Traditional doctors in some western medical science, establishing research institutes were all part of the Great Leap period. Insisting Traditional doctors be hired in western-style hospitals and that western doctors receive Traditional education can be seen as part of the Red versus Expert campaign.

The latest strategy of the Party is to promote combined treatment.

A number of these action strategies lost sight of some of Mao's original comments on integration. While he called for a 'United Front' of the two schools, he also said that western doctors should 'take responsibility' for improving Traditional medicine with modern science; that they should 'help, stimulate and reform' it, that they should organize, upgrade and utilize those of the old school that 'can be used'.

Little in the study tour material indicates the emergence of a 'United Front'. Observations suggest Traditional medicine and practitioners play a subordinate role today in the PRC health care system. Statements by western physicians reflect commitment to integration or at least, use of selected Traditional medicine but on their own terms and in a context of limited western pharmaceuticals.

Western medicine, western bio-medical science and western trained physicians continue to dominate the unique health care system of the People's Republic of China. But they have been forced to share their policy-making and implementation power to the extent that a medical tradition, which had not been able to hold up to scientific scrutiny in theoretical and diagnostic terms, is being absorbed into medical treatment. Individual citizens, western physicians and medical educators, hospital administrators, Barefoot Doctors and other health practitioners all have accepted the utilization of myriad Traditional treatments for an unusually wide variety of illness and disease conditions.

Despite enormous political pressure over a thirty-year period for greater enthusiasm and broader utilization of Traditional medicine, western doctors resisted in the name of the world culture of modern bio-medical science to which the medical profession everywhere owes strong allegiance and loyalty. Neither the widely accepted realities of economic necessity nor the political obligations of an enormously powerful leader of a rural revolution nor the power struggle of a successful Communist Party to gain dominance over recalcitrant elites could shake the hold of western bio-medical science. Ironically, it could well be scientific research itself that finally secures a future place for a very old medicine which not too many years ago seemed a medical curiosity.

Some Americans, rightfully dissatisfied with aspects of the American health care system, have romanticized the PRC health care system including Traditional medicine and in the process, lose some perspectives on realities. There is very much to be admired about the system, its remarkable innovations and remarkable accomplishments, without blurring its actual nature. Suggestions that Traditional medicine is or should be practiced in its entirety (Porkert 1978) or that the Chinese are now backing away from the exciting model of health care delivery they originally gave the world (Rifkin 1979) ignores certain realities including the original policy motivations. It ignores the pragmatic realities if practicing medicine on a day-to-day basis. And it ignores the persistence of that ubiquitous characteristic of all social institutions: change. It also fails to make the important distinction between stated policy and its actual implementation.

Mao wanted Traditional medicine 'made scientific'. Efforts proceed in this direction. Mao called for western physicians to bring Traditional medicine into the twentieth century. They now work in the same institutions albeit not as a 'Unified Front'. And the two groups remain apart organizationally. What this will mean is unclear. Nonetheless, Mao's political and economic needs and strategies have given Chung-i new life. And if it makes meaningful and substantiated contributions to common and chronic illness, to the treatment of acute abdomines and to prevention, then Mao's new Chinese Medicine will be, as he hoped, a significant contribution to world medical culture. The PRC is certainly commanding world-wide attention because of the integration.

Economic necessity may continue to be a strong motivation as some knowledgeable observers (Study Journal 1979) suggest that the improvement of the health care system will not be a high priority in the next decade or two. Early rural political obligations may have now been satisfied as well as the desire to enhance cultural pride. In fact, cultural pride may now insist, in a new scientific age when kindergarten children are taught to sing songs entitled 'We Love Science' that Traditional medicine be more rigorously legitimized with scientific research. As for the Red versus Expert battle, it appears to be the Experts' turn for resurgence and active participation in the modernization process.

What has politics wrought? A remarkable accomplishment: Traditional medicine, preserved in part, and actively utilized as it is assimilated into western medical practice; Mao Tse-tung very much vindicated in his astute politics, astute economics and astute understanding of power in medical settings.

For political reasons, Mao forced a most peculiar policy onto the health care system of the People's Republic of China. This should force us to reflect, anew, on the essentially political nature of health policy and all health care systems. The PRC, facing problems of personnel shortages and maldistribution (both found in western industrialized health care systems as well) met the resistance, dominance and power of the medical profession with a dramatic political counterforce such as no other national group of physicians has faced. It took such a force both to push a typically resistant dominant profession, and to circumvent them. The goal, to preserve and modernize a scientifically rejected medical tradition, was an incredible one given modern scientific values, but by 1981 it seems at least partially in process. By the same token, the ability of a powerful, high status profession to both bend to great pressure yet remain resilient enough to survive repeated attacks and stay in command is equally incredible.

This deserves special attention in examination of the larger issue of the intrinsically political character of all health care systems and the continuing ability of physicians as a group to maintain power and protect their interests in a variety of systems: unplanned, nationalized, socialized, or rationalized.

NOTES

1. Like most material gathered during study tours to the People's Republic of China, this is based on translations by China International Travel Services guides. These hardworking people carry out their task most conscientiously but with technical subjects like health care, errors can easily occur. Other problems of distortion are possible as well. However, conscientiously taken notes as well as cassette recordings were carefully transcribed to create a 230-page group journal of all briefings and discussion sessions.

2. This observation was made during a briefing with Ambassador Leonard Woodcock at the American Embassy in Beijing, August 1979.

REFERENCES

Croizier, R. C.
1965 Traditional Medicine in Communist China: Science, Communism and Cultural Nationalism. China Quarterly 5.
1968 Traditional Medicine in Modern China. Harvard University Press, Cambridge.
Gordon S., and Allan T.
1952 The Scalpel and the Sword: The Story of Doctor Norman Bethune. Monthly Review Press, New York.
Horn J. S.
1969 Away with All Pests. An English Surgeon in People's Republic of China: 1954–1969. Monthly Review Press, New York.
Kleinman A.
1978 Traditional Medicine in China. Chapter in the report of the Rural Health Systems Delegation of the Committee on Scholarly Communication with the People's Republic of China. (June).
Lampton, D.
1977 The Politics of Medicine in China. Westview Press, Boulder, Colorado.
1980 Personal Correspondence.
Porkert M.
1978 The Theoretical Formulations of Chinese Medicine: Systems of Correspondence. MIT Press, Cambridge, Ma.
Rifkin S.
1979 Health Care in China: The Experts take Command. University of Hong Kong, August. Unpublished manuscript.
Sidel, V.
1973 Serve the People: Observations on Medicine in the People's Republic of China. The Macy Foundation, New York.
Study Journal
1979 Study Journal of The University of Michigan/Michigan State University Health Care Study Tour to the People's Republic of China. Unpublished manuscript, available from the author upon request.

3
RURAL HEALTH CARE DELIVERY IN THE PEOPLE'S REPUBLIC OF CHINA: IS IT EQUITABLY DISTRIBUTED?

with Paul Pongor

INTRODUCTION

One of the first responses to early descriptions of the health care delivery system of the People's Republic of China was that it represented a more appropriate model for developing nations than that typically exported by western nations.

The western model is focused on using specialized personnel in a comparatively sophisticated health service to deliver the necessary health care. The ideal, presumably, is to expand these services until the entire population is covered, an ideal seldom attained. As a result of this approach, however, facilities tend to be centered in the urban areas of a nation, predominantly curative in nature and providing services to a relatively small group of the population. One obvious explanation for this pattern is that the limited resources generally available to a developing nation restricts the expansion of the health system in its rural areas.

An alternate approach is personified by that which has evolved in the People's Republic of China. This has been described as community-based or essentially primary health

Portions of this material were delivered at a symposium: "Political Process and the Health Care System of the People's Republic of China," Society for Applied Anthropology, Denver, Colorado, March, 1980.

care which focuses on the dvelopmental needs of the most deprived populations, those in rural areas. This approach to health policy emphasizes local initiative, the utilization of the least expensive personnel, techniques, material and the goal of minimal organization to deal with patients as well as improve the living conditions of the community's inhabitants. The focus is on combining curative with preventive, promotive, rehabilitative, and community development activities (Djukanovic 1975).

The history, the health policy evolution and descriptions of this health system are now well-known to American readers but only in a superficial manner. This paper, based on observations of the rural health care delivery system in the PRC in 1979 and 1981 will provide case studies of contrasting rural facilities and the networks within which they are immersed as well as a comparison with urban health networks. These case studies can help bring into focus the factors that influence and modify PRC health care delivery in the grassroots. The promulgation and idealization of the Chinese model must be tempered with a more realistic understanding of how national health policy emerges as it confronts the practical exigences of implementation in the countryside.

Historical Synopsis of Health Care Delivery in the PRC

A very quick summary of rural health care delivery in the PRC. The first modern government in China, the Republican and the Nationalists Periods (1911–1949) attempted to address rural health care issues but with meager resources and fragmented effort interrupted by civil war, World War II and overwhelming political and economic problems. During the Republican period, there was an effort to begin a plan for comprehensive rural health, the cornerstone of which was to be county hospitals (Lampton 1974:1). This never proceeded beyond the establishment of a few models. The medical manpower pool was a meager one. Western-style physicians ranged from 2,919 registered in 1932 to estimates of from 10,000 to 41,400 in 1949 when the Chinese Communists took over the government (Croizier 1973:4) and these practiced primarily in urban areas. There were large numbers of Traditional doctors including bone-setters, herbalists, and acupuncturists in the rural areas but absence of any well-defined national standards produced a wide variety of backgrounds and skills with most inadequately trained even by Traditional medicine standards (Croizier 1973:4).

The experience of the CCP Army during the 1930s and 1940s produced some health care innovations shaped by desperate need and desperate lack of resources. Despite the Red Army doctors disdain for Traditional medicine and its practitioners, Traditional approaches were emphasized and peasants trained as para-medics. The Army also organized local communities for primitive health campaigns. All of these efforts were the forerunners of approaches to rural health care that have become famous in the PRC today.

With the Chinese Communist Party assuming power in 1949, these early experiments in health care delivery became national policy. In 1950, under Mao's direction, the First National Health Congress was held and from it came the dictum that health work should serve the masses (New China Monthly 1950:166). Two basic health units were reconstructed at the meeting: (1) the Epidemic Prevention Stations from which the early rural health care structure emerged. Their major responsibility was communicable disease reporting, innoculation campaigns, dealing with sanitation problems in their area and carrying out public health work. (2) Affiliated Clinics to provide medical care and to carry out health programs for local people. Health manpower was to be gradually increased through accelerated enrollments in medical schools, utilization of para-professionals and the legitimization of Traditional doctors. Mass campaigns, against specific health problems, called "Patriotic Health Campaigns" were first initiated in 1952. Their purpose was to improve village water sanitation and to eradicate the "four pests": rats, flies, mosquitoes, and bedbugs.

Despite Mao's rural policy emphasis, implementation seemed to stress the development of the urban health system. During the 1950s and early 1960s some of China's efforts in health care were copied from models seen in other countries especially the Soviet Union (Rifkin 1973:143). Initially, the Ministry of Health was organized using a model provided by the USSR Ministry of Health. The Chinese Ministry of Health also seemed to use Soviet strategies. Its first Five-Year Plan

(1953–1957) only mentioned that "... sanitation work in rural districts must be gradually improved." However, "In health and medical services, priority must be given to improving the work in industrial [urban] areas ..." (Djukanovik and Mach 1975:37).

With the drive to collectivize the countryside during the 1950s "Great Leap Forward," promises of a rural network of health care delivery became even more pressing. The existence of local medical units would make the commune system more attractive to the rural citizenry and be tangible evidence of the Chinese Communist Party's commitment to their well-being. Progress was slow and reports of the inadequacy of rural health care resources persisted into the 1960s. The Great Leap Forward paradoxically forced the rural health care system into a real dilemma. With the Great Leap Forward came an elimination of all fees at the time of treatment. Predictably, health care costs skyrocketed upward and imposed even greater problems upon the already financially strapped rural system.

Increasing costs, along with other political and economic problems, lead to a decrease in brigade cooperative health funds. The result was a cutback in available services with the eventual erosion of free (collectively-run) commune clinics (Lampton 1974:19). It is not surprising then to hear reports of peasants having to "... journey over hilly areas and cross rivers to see a doctor or buy medicine" and after arriving at their destination, they were "discriminated against," shown indifference or "even rejected by hospitals" (Orleans 1977:25). The inadequate care being delivered to China's masses laid the groundwork, on the eve of the Cultural Revolution, for Mao's 19 June 1965 directive: "In medical and health work ... put the stress on the rural areas" (Gordon 1973:70), reflecting the continued frustration in delivering care to the peasants. His directive paved the way for the institutionalization of the Barefoot Doctor program as well as establishing the policy of sending urban physicians out to the rural countryside to practice and teach health care. It also accelerated the organization of delivery units at all levels of the rural political and economic structure. But this historical sketch indicates that implementation of health policy has not always been easy and as the following indicates, implementation has by no means been equitable.

Out in the Countryside

The rural health and medical system as we observed it in 1979 and 1981 is basically a county five-tier system. This is in contrast to the three or four tiers usually described in the literature (Mechanic and Kleinman 1980:63; Rifkin 1973:146; Sidel 1973:88). The first tier, staffed primarily by the Barefoot Doctor and assisted by midwives and health aides, is the production brigade health station. It is at this level where the peasant often first comes into contact with the medical system. If the patient's problem is beyond the scope of the station, the patient is ideally referred up to the next level of the system, the commune hospital. Staffed with western-style and Traditional doctors, nurses and other health workers and sometimes with a limited number of in-patient beds, the commune hospital is equipped to handle somewhat more difficult cases.[1] The third level of the system is a more sophisticated commune hospital known as the District (or Central) Commune Hospital which serves its own commune and four to six others by offering specialized services.[2] The fourth tier is the County Hospital which is the most elaborate of the strictly rural facilities. And according to our information, the County Bureaus of Public Health are emerging as a fifth tier in the system, clearly functioning on the health rather than medical side of the system but with increasing responsibility for managing the entire county health care system (Figure 3.1).

What these county systems look like, however, varies greatly around the country. Among the counties we visited in 1979 was one in an area never before observed by foreigners where there was a significant emphasis on Traditional approaches and heavy demands made on relatively limited facilities. In significant contrast was a rural county observed in 1981 with an almost exclusively western-style orientation, well developed and expanding facilities, excellent state financial support yet providing essentially the same level of care. In addition, we observed commune health facilities in geographically diverse areas both rural and suburban that reflected additional contrasts in how the PRC rural health care system has actually emerged. These descriptive case histories can be compared with a summary of other counties and communes that have been reported in the literature. From this will emerge a highly varied pattern of health care development and the social factors that have influenced health policy as it has actually been implemented.

COUNTY LEVEL: CASE STUDY OF NONG AN COUNTY HOSPITAL

The enormous crowds of people on the streets outside Nong An County Hospital seemed to corroborate our guide's contention that we were the first foreigners to visit this location in decades (Study Journal 1979:178). This heightened our interest even further in the history and description of the hospital, its services, staff and the health problems it attempts to address.

History and General Description

Located approximately forty miles from Chang Chun in Kirin province, Nong An hospital serves a county population of 960,000 which is primarily rural, living on 5,400 hectares of farmland and in two towns of which Nong An Town is one (with a population of 60,000). Throughout the county there are thirty communes and 350 production brigades. The county hospital is linked with these units in a health care network that includes district commune hospitals, commune health centers and production brigade health clinics. The hospital apparently existed in some form before the Revolution as it was described as being "liberated in 1948." It was, however, in a much less developed form as it only saw out-patients, had a "low level of technology" and a staff of five doctors. But, we were told that "under Chairman Mao, the hospital developed very quickly."

Our hosts stated that the hospital "reports to the County Public Health Bureau and is under the leadership of the Branch Committee of the Chinese Communist Party." We were also told that its guiding principles are to "put prevention first," to serve the workers and the peasants, to unite the

Chinese doctors with the western doctors (and that "this is now being taken very seriously"). Finally, that by combining medical work with the national (revolutionary) movement these last thirty years, the county's health has been greatly changed. These principles are those articulated by Chairman Mao in 1950 at the first National Health Conference in Beijing. Working under these principles, we were told that the plague, polio, smallpox and diphtheria have been eliminated and "some of the recurrent diseases brought under control."

Organization

The hospital's organization includes a medical school for nurses and Barefoot Doctors (currently enrolling 100 students); 350 in-patient beds and nine in-patient departments; a variety of out-patient services and an herb garden. See Figure 3.2 for a review of hospital services.

The hospital also supervises four health stations out in the countryside for TB, prevention of seasonal disease and cholera. They are engaged in various forms of research, primarily observational studies on pneumonial bronchitis and "common" diseases. An emergency car is available to transport patients with serious illness and those with emergencies are admitted immediately. There may be a four to five day wait for others.

A tour of selected departments in the hospital permitted a glimpse of the equipment in use. For example, the X-ray equipment we saw was made in Shanghai in 1933, the dental clinic equipment was also from that decade. The major equipment noted in the Emergency Room was an oxygen tank and IV poles.

The primary health problems found in the ER and treated in this hospital are factory injuries, pneumonia, heart attack and gastric distress. Other adult problems are bronchitis (during the winter), kidney inflammation and arthritis. The major pediatric problem is infant pneumonia. In 1978, 1,200 children ages one to five were admitted for this condition of which twenty-four died. The following statistics were provided:

Patient Population	Treatment Results
4,906 In-patients (6 months in 1979)	86 percent cured 11.5 percent feeling better .5 percent transferred 1.8 percent mortality
Out-patients 800 daily	

Personnel

"Medical workers" (294) include ninety-six western-style doctors, nine Traditional doctors and 140 nurses. They have some supervisory responsibility for the commune district hospitals which are staffed by approximately twenty western-style doctors, and the commune health centers which may have eight to twelve doctors. Overall, there are 400 western-style doctors in the county. (An interesting aside is that fifty-three of these, or 13 percent, are members of the Chinese Communist Party). Eighty of the physicians are graduates of medical universities and the rest received medical college training. Ten percent have done or are doing post-graduate work at Norman Bethune Medical University in the closest major city, Chang Chun. The county hospital itself has continuous in-service training. Currently three medical professors from the city and seven university medical students are at the hospital as consultants.

Use of Traditional Medicine

Although the number of Traditional doctors at the County Hospital was proportionately small, we were told that extensive use is made of Traditional medicine and techniques. An acupuncture treatment room with electric equipment serves both in- and out-patient needs. Acupuncture is used to treat appendicitis, gall stones, ectopic pregnancies, brain hemorrhages and infant pneumonia with a reported 90 percent success rate. The treatment also includes herbal medicines. For example, in 296 successful cases of appendicitis studied at the hospital, 187 were treated in the western-style with surgery and 109 with Traditional medicine.

The hospital grows, dries, stores and manufactures its own Traditional medicine from a three mos herb garden attached to the central building. Two-hundred seventeen different herbs are grown here, tended by a Traditional doctor who is assisted by all the medical and hospital staff on a rotating basis. The garden is also used for educational purposes to instruct western doctors and Barefoot Doctors during their Traditional medicine studies.

Such study groups are regularly given at the county hospital both for in-service training and for doctors who come from the countryside. By the same token, Traditional doctors receive western training to improve their "technological skills so that they will be able to perform simple operations."

During a tour of the garden various herbs were pointed out and their uses described. For example, the "double flower herb" is often utilized for the "effective" treatment of inflammation, infant pneumonia and bone infection.

Acupuncture anesthesia is utilized for thyroidectomies and difficult labor deliveries.

Financial Information

Patients coming to the hospital have insurance provided either by the government or their factories. This, we are told, is true of 90 percent of the patients. Those 10 percent from the rural areas are paid for by their brigade cooperative medical plans. Elderly are treated free and anyone else not covered "can apply for admission." The 10 percent rural figure is an interesting reflection of the number of patients presumably referred up from the commune levels. We would be able to make the following approximate calculations: 4,906 patients in six months x 2 = 9,812 − 10% = 981 rural patients out of a possible rural population (960,000 − 120,000: approximate population of two towns) of 840,000 or less than 1 percent of the rural population using the county hospital.

The total budget for the county hospital in 1978 was 600,000 Yuan and was paid by the State (central government). The average monthly salary for all personnel is 60 Yuan and the highest is 150 Yuan. We were told that this last figure applied to the highest for any administrator, western or Traditional doctor or nurse. An average day in this hospital costs 2.50 Yuan. There seemed to be considerable pride in how the use of herbal medicines keep costs down. In this context we were told that an appendicitis case treated with herbs cost five Yuan while the operation cost thirty Yuan.

Summary

Overall, this example of a facility on the county level reveals a hospital that expanded impressively between 1949 and 1979, now offering a large array of secondary level facilities. It is sophisticated enough to provide educational services. Its in-patient services are reasonable. Noteworthy is the frugality coming with a heavy reliance on Traditional treatment. Major financial support comes from the central government level with additional revenue generated from several different insurance systems. Ties to the urban health system are through in-service continuing education for the hospital staff. Ties to the commune network are primarily through para-professional and nursing education. This hospital, however, serves a surprisingly small proportion of rural peasants.

YE COUNTY AND ITS HOSPITAL

During a study tour in 1981, an opportunity was provided to visit another county and its hospital. This had strikingly different characteristics and appeared to represent a significantly different model of development.

At first introduction, Ye County did not look particularly different from other rural areas we had visited. Its fields appear fruitful and well-tended. Some of the villages we were told, dated back four-hundred years. Transportation on the roads was the usual mix of trucks and donkey carts. Its major crops are maize, wheat and peanuts and 94 percent of the population work in agriculture. Running water is available to approximately 6 percent of the population, although there are 80,300 hand pumps. There has been a significant improvement in the 142,800 latrines in various areas of the rural county. They are no longer built so near the pigsties. And there have been some other significant improvements as well: infant mortality in 1948 was 132/1,000; in 1980 that figure was 11.7/1,000. In 1948, average life expectancy was forty-five; in 1980, it was seventy-two for males and seventy-seven for females. Ye is purported to have one of the most effective birth planning programs in the PRC. In point of fact, this county in Shandong Province, has become a World Health Organization model for the study of effective rural health care delivery. Its statistics have been verified, its approaches are being carefully studied. Once a year the WHO and Ye County Public Health Bureau run a two-week course for health workers from other locations in the PRC itself, analyzing and teaching Ye County's approach to health care delivery.

Ye is perhaps one of the few places in the world where the developmental level is agricultural and the health status statistics are industrial. A remarkable accomplishment.

Its total county population is 827,500 divided into twenty-seven communes, 1,010 Production Brigades, 4,080 Production Teams; all-in-all 195,000 households. It has several bustling market towns, one of which (Yen Tai) contains the County hospital. This hospital was a strikingly more sophisticated facility than its counterpart in Nong An. Not only was it more elaborately developed and better financed, but it was part of a much more extensive network of facilities. Yet it served a smaller population than Nong An but with a budget proportionately almost the same.

A description of Ye County Hospital, its various departments, units and statistical information is included at the end of this chapter (Figure 3.3).

The most prominent difference, compared to Nong An County Hospital, is the almost total absence of Traditional medicine, Traditional approaches and Traditional personnel. There is no herb garden, no herbal medicine preparation room, only one Traditional doctor and no known effort to train younger practitioners in this mode. One-third of the western-style doctors have, however, studied some Traditional medicine. The one practicing Traditional doctor does have his own out-patient clinic and his own ward, suggesting quite a segregated environment. Ye County Hospital seemed almost entirely western in orientation.

Another major difference must be noted: the much greater percentage of rural patients served at Ye County Hospital. Eighty percent of out-patients are rural and 90 percent of the in-patients. This is in dramatic contrast to the Nong An figures. How might this be interpreted? Several explanations suggest themselves: that Ye County Hospital enjoys a better reputation; that a referral network with the lower level rural facilities is better developed and integrated; that lower level commune hospitals are better able to pay the cost of referrals from their medical funds and therefore make more referrals; that individual peasants are better able to pay on their own when they circumvent the commune level. While no assertion can be made with certainty, the comparison strongly suggests the impact of economic factors. A more affluent rural hospital moves more towards a western-style model and enjoys a better reputation among its potential consumers.

It can also be seen that the Ye County Public Health Bureau itself is a more elaborate organization with direct responsibilities for a variety of services which appear under the hospital in Nong An.

Based on information provided at the two county hospitals, statistics are compared and contrasted in Table 3.1 at the end of this chapter.

If all the figures are accurate and trustworthy (we must admit to some skepticism about Nong An's "success rates" and salary scale), the following observations may be made about these two rural county hospitals. Proportionate to population, Ye County spends slightly less, has half the number of beds, a faster bed turnover rate, slightly higher bed occupancy, and a lower number of hospital visits per person. It also has a lower doctor/bed ratio and a much lower nurse/bed ratio (this is most likely a reflection of the nurses' school at Nong An). It also has less than half the number of western-style doctors and only one

Traditional doctor to Nong An's nine. Also noteworthy (although the implications are not clear) is that it has a higher percentage of doctors who are members of the Chinese Communist Party. Of greatest interest are the disease patterns it confronts. For adults, it shades towards an industrial nation while Nong An is more conventionally agriculture. For children, the agricultural pattern is present in both. Overall, however, Ye County Hospital emerges as making much more efficient use of its resources and as emphasizing a much more distinctly western model.

Ye County hospital and Nong An County hospital can be compared, in a variety of ways, to other county hospitals described in the literature (Table 3.2). Obviously, we must recognize the different years these facilities were written up. When the raw figures are all rendered proportionate to population, Ye County emerges as significantly ahead in all dimensions. All explanations for this are simply not available, but a clearly successful agricultural area has both concentrated its own resources on its health care system and attracted heavy financial support from the central government as well.

It may be reasoned that our study tours in 1979 and 1980 were shown rural facilities that the authorities deemed acceptable for foreign visitors. This is probably true for all visitors to the country; therefore descriptions to date represent the "best" and no reports provide insight into the weakest elements in the rural health delivery system. Yet, from what has been seen, at least two different models emerge probably exemplified by Nong An County and Ye County. These may be designated as a "Traditional Model" and a "Western Model," the major differentiating factor being reliance on Traditional medicine and approaches, and the major determinant being economics.

MULTI-COMMUNE LEVEL: CASE STUDY OF KAIAN COMMUNE DISTRICT (CENTRAL) HOSPITAL

An organizational strategy that has been tried in a number of areas in connection with the commune hospitals or centers is the use of a central hospital. A central hospital not only provides referral services for the production brigades in the immediate area surrounding the hospital but also provides supervision to other, less sophisticated commune hospitals in the area and receives referrals from these hospitals. Thus, the central hospital assumes a position in a tier between the commune hospital and the county hospital. It may have a particularly important in-patient function since commune hospitals or centers often do not have in-patient beds.

Organization

KaiAn commune, with a population of 29,782, has twelve production brigades and 126 production teams. The central district hospital in the KaiAn People's Commune is responsible for five or six communes situated in the surrounding area as well as its own commune. Two-hundred square meters large, this seventy-two room, fifty-one bed hospital is staffed by forty-three medical personnel in addition to forty-nine Barefoot Doctors, and attempts to meet both the out-patient and in-patient needs of the area. The hospital also contains a pharmacy, medical laboratory, an X-ray room, a cardiograph room, surgical facilities and can also make medications for the hospital's use from Chinese medicinal herbs grown in a garden adjacent to the hospital containing some 310 different plant species.

This unit directs various mass movements commonly used to prevent and eliminate certain diseases like diphtheria. In addition, the hospital does work in the area of obstetrics, gynecology and family planning. They also perform much of the dental work for the immediate area as well as participate in the health propaganda work commonly used in China to educate the Chinese people about some of the more basic aspects of medicine. The KaiAn District Hospital participates in the training of Barefoot Doctors who work in the surrounding area with the Barefoot Doctors journeying to the hospital and holding meetings to discuss the medical work they are required to perform at their brigade. The district has a BFD ratio of 1:607. (See Figure 3.4).

Herb Garden and Use of Traditional Medicine

The hospital herb garden was started quite recently, in 1975. A seventy-year old Traditional doctor is in charge of the garden which contains plants grown locally, transplanted from other rural and mountain areas and even imported from abroad. According to Mechanic and Kleinman (1980) this is a new development in post-Liberation China as previously, herbs were highly localized. This herb garden director earns seventy-five Yuan a month, a salary usually earned by the average western-style doctor. Production brigades also have their own herb gardens with each specializing in seven different plants. The hospital manufactures 160 different kinds of medicines from its home-grown herbs with the medical laboratory analyzing the pills that are produced and utilizing "control for quality." It was possible to view the pill-making room and a simple hand-operated machine that formed the dried and crushed herbs into small, round tablets.

This activity provides some insight into the economic constraints of intermediate-level rural health care. While KaiAn Commune is well supported by a medical cooperative sickness insurance fund (20 percent of the rural areas are not financially able to establish such funds), frugality is practiced by reducing the purchase of expensive western-style pharmaceuticals. During a visit to the hospital Injection Room, the information on western pharmaceuticals was that vaccinations are available for cholera, measles, encephalitis, diphtheria, whooping cough, TB and polio. Outside of these western vaccines, "the strongest medicine dispensed is penicillin."

The pharmacy contained two rooms; one for herbal medicines, one for western. Four-hundred Traditional medicines are stocked. Three health workers are assigned to duty here and one is the herbalist who has forty years of experience which began when he was apprenticed at age ten. He is responsible for teaching the younger workers.

Selected Services

A further picture of the kind of care delivered at such an intermediate tier of the rural delivery system emerged as we visited a dental room, maternity room, and surgery.

The dental room contained a chair and drilling equipment common in the USA in the 1930s. The dental worker was a graduate of Harbin Medical College (a Chinese educational institution that trains secondary doctors and medical assistants of various sorts). It was also said that she was apprenticed to an "old master."

The maternity room dispenses both obstetrical and family planning services. In 1978 the hospital delivered 340 babies and performed eighty abortions under the direction of a female maternity doctor who graduated from a medical school. However, 80 percent of the babies in the area were delivered at home attended by Barefoot Doctors. A family planning chart adorned the walls, bearing the following information for 1977–1978:

3,468 women of child-bearing age: 520 are sterilized;

2,389 have IUDs. 12.8 birth rate; 6.91 rate of natural increase (Study Journal, 1979).

The family planning service provides various contraceptive devices that included pills and condoms as well as those listed on the chart. An important responsibility was to promote family planning discussions among commune couples to attempt to set family target goals in conjunction with State population goals.

A visit to the surgery room revealed a small room with limited equipment. The kinds of operations performed at this level of care included: ulcers, appendicitis, hernia, sterilizations. Chest and heart surgery was referred to the county hospital. Three to five operations were scheduled per week or about 200 a year, performed by a surgeon with five years of training at a medical university. Barefoot Doctors assist in the surgery. Local drug anesthesia is utilized. The equipment in the room included ultra-violet light to create a sterile field over the operating table and an autoclave for sterilizing instruments.

Financial Information

Some information about the finances of this district hospital was available. The annual budget includes 20,000 Yuan primarily for wages, while the County Bureau of Health supplies all of the equipment for the facility. The cooperative medical service costs each peasant thirty to sixty fen (average annual peasant salary 325 Yuan[3] (Tsui 1979). The rest of the cost is paid by the production brigade although it is acceptable for rich brigades to pay more than poor ones. The following examples were given:

Rich Brigades: Yuan 1.5 per year per person by the
 Brigade; 60 fen paid by the individual member
Poor Brigades: Yuan 1.0 per year per person by the
 Brigade; 30 fen paid by the individual member
All patients pay 5 fen per visit.

KaiAn and Other Central (District) Hospitals

KaiAn can be compared to two other central or district commune hospitals reported in the literature (Table 3.3). The information is rather fragmented but does reflect that KaiAn compares favorably with both a suburban and another rural facility. We were unable to visit a district commune hospital in Ye County but we know that there are four in the system and that they are directly supervised by the county hospital. Furthermore, referral figures indicate that there is a close relationship between the units indicating a national utilization pattern that at least reflects an efficient bureaucratic structure. Such efficiency does not appear evident in Nong An and therefore suggests the possibility of wide variation in how well county systems work.

Commune Hospitals

In 1979 and 1981, the study groups visited a total of four commune hospitals, three of them were suburban and were less than one-half hour from a major metropolitan area;

only one was rather rusticated. Our visits included MaLu Commune in the suburbs of Shanghai which is really a well-developed small town in its own right with a diversified economy, Shin Hua outside of Canton, a popular commune on the "tourist circuit" and one which has been reported a number of times in the research literature; the 5th May Commune in suburban Shenyang with a thriving mixed economy that had just permitted the installation of running water to all homes; Ye Commune in affluent Ye County which has already been described. Every place we saw, therefore, was among the best developed communes, those thought appropriate for foreign scrutiny. (Figures 3.5 through 3.8 provide information for each of these four commune hospitals).

It is clear to see that they all conform to a similar pattern of organization and all have a formal relationship to the delivery units below them. All take responsibility for BFD training. There are some noteworthy differences in BFD/ population ratios as well as medical worker/population ratios. The more rural Ye County has a heavier reliance on BFDs while the two closest to major cities have a much better medical worker/population ratio. We also found the most sophisticated medical equipment (ultra-sound) in the Canton suburbs. Furthermore, some of these commune hospitals had herb gardens or seemed to rely as heavily on Traditional medicines as the Nong An and KaiAn facilities which were at higher levels.

A quick comparison between the 5th May and KaiAn District Hospital (serving five communes: both visited in 1979) indicates the following:

(1) 5th May serves only one commune but has one-third more medical workers
than KaiAn;

(2) 5th May has ninety Barefoot Doctors to KaiAn's forty-nine, almost twice as many;

(3) 5th May offers almost precisely the same array of medical services.

While it is true that 5th May has a one-third larger population, KaiAn serves additional communes so that several significant ratios are skewed in the suburban commune's favor. 5th May, closer to a large city and wealthier than the more remote KaiAn, appears to have better facilities for fewer people with less relative need because of close urban facilities.

When all the reports on Shin Hua are put together, a rare ten-year portrait of this commune and its health facilities emerges (see Table 3.4). Despite the fragmentary nature of the information in some years, we can observe a 40 percent increase in budget between 1972 and 1981 but only a 11 percent increase in population. There was also a 70 percent increase in medical workers and a 70 percent increase in number of BFDs and a BFD/population ratio that went from 1:1,722 to 1:514. The total medical worker/population ratio went from 1:1377 to 1:724. While one may guess that Shin Hua has been considered a show place for the Canton area, it can be documented that significant improvements have taken place in the decade since 1971.

FOUR-COMMUNE COMPARISONS

When we compare the four communes on various dimensions (where parallel information is available) the major difference noted in Table 3.5 is an inverse relationship between BFD/population and medical workers/population with the more rural areas relying more on less trained personnel. Observationally speaking, the vintage and sophistication of equipment was better at MaLu and Shin Hua and these rely less on Traditional medicine and practitioners. Shin Hua has ultrasound equipment, one of the first signs of high technology we saw. (Several hospital directors in urban facilities did remark that they would like ultrasound and CT scanners). MaLu commune hospital had no X-ray or surgical facilities because these, and their two surgeons recently moved to the County hospital so they will no longer provide those kinds of services. An informant at Shin Hua did admit that during droughts, the brigades suspended their contributions to the coop medical plans but tried to make it up during a good harvest. This is a question that is rarely asked and would be a good indicator of the stability and financial solvency of commune medical services. It was surprising that Shin Hua, the most affluent commune visited should have a health care system still vulnerable to agricultural exigencies.

SOCIAL FACTORS INFLUENCING THE RURAL SYSTEM

One of the most extensive studies of rural health facilities in the People's Republic of China can be found in an unpublished manuscript (1979) by Tsui Wai-Ying, from the Chinese University of Hong Kong. She corroborates the regionalized nature of the rural health care system and reiterates that facilities are related through a chain of units from the simplest at the production brigade level (the cooperative medical clinics) to the commune health centers, to the district commune hospitals (serving several communes) to the county hospital and attached facilities. These are the basic units of the rural system and are the level through which a patient passes who needs increasingly sophisticated medical care.

According to this author, while local autonomy of these units has been emphasized, there is developing a move to strengthen the links between the county health bureau and the whole commune health delivery system.

Tsui's paper, which reports the details of an in-depth study of two rural communes and their health facilities, posits two major external factors which correlate with the degree to which the health care system of a commune is developed. She calls those factors "geographic access" and "economic access." By this she suggests that communes will be capable of different health care services used on proximity to urban centers and relative to their particular income levels. Lampton (1978) suggests the same thing based on his observations and assessments.

Her own study concludes that richer communes, closer to urban centers will have better, more extensive facilities with better trained and more personnel. She points out that this is contrary to national health policy that mandates equal access to good care throughout the nation. She suggests that more remote, poorer communes will require heavy State subsidy in order to fulfill State policy.

Our own observations corroborate these findings. This has been demonstrated in the comparisons of the county hospitals and the commune hospitals, including one district (or central) commune hospital. Despite the fact that all sites visited were considered acceptable for visitors to see, clear disparities and inequities could be observed. One may reasonably surmise that even greater differences could be substantiated if a random sample of rural health facilities could be viewed.

BY CONTRAST: AN URBAN HEALTH CARE NETWORK

One may grasp the PRC health care system a bit better by looking at urban health facilities.

An extended briefing with a Harbin Municipal Public Health Bureau staff enables us to render a detailed picture of an urban health care delivery system and the way in which city officials view their ties to rural facilities (Journal 1979:169).

Harbin is one of the major metropolitan areas of Northeast China encompassing a population of 2.3 million. Its urban health network includes 650 medical care establishments, 14,546 hospital beds, 28,457 medical workers of different types and 2,515 Barefoot Doctors and health aides in the immediately surrounding rural areas. Table 3.6 demonstrates the tremendous gaps between this city and our four rural communes.

The Deputy Director of the Public Health Bureau described the system as having four levels. The first is a combination of provincial and municipal level institutions. The second level in the services provided in Harbin's seven districts throughout which the provincial and municipal hospital are spread. He described the third level as the commune level, suggesting that commune hospital centers and district hospitals are linked officially to the urban system. The fourth level is the Neighborhood Health Care Center Station. Also on the fourth level are the production brigade health stations. This urban system is depicted in Figure 3.9.

The briefing stated explicitly that the surrounding rural area was part of the urban health system and linked on both the commune hospital and the production brigade cooperative medical clinic levels. No mention was made, however, of links to the county hospital or the county public health bureau. This is an area for further investigation. Either no specific links exist or county hospitals are not as important in a rural area, which is so close to extensive municipal facilities, as they are in remote rural areas. Our Harbin informants emphatically referred to commune-level care as being integrated into the municipality's system both at the hospital and production brigade level. It is particularly interesting to note that one of the municipal neighborhood health stations is specifically designated to work with the rural production brigade stations.

The impact of these urban-rural linkages is not altogether clear from currently available information. However, in a condition of limited economic resources for all aspects of the Chinese health care system, both rural and urban, the links may represent a symbiotic relationship that both strengthens the rural system and weakens the urban one.

Several observers have commented on the general economic context of the system. Robert Blendon, in a recent issue of the *New England Journal of Medicine* (1979) presents a closely reasoned analysis suggesting that economic priorities in the PRC have not, to date, permitted a particular emphasis on the health care system. The reliance everywhere on herbal medicines, no doubt, is motivated as much by financial considerations as by ideological ones, particularly in the countryside. While the uses of herbal treatments were described in large city hospitals, the herbal garden attached to Nong An County hospital and the even larger one at the commune district hospital suggests an even heavier reliance and use in the countryside.

During a briefing at the American Embassy, Ambassador Woodcock also proferred the opinion that under China's current leadership the health care system would be a relatively low priority (Study Journal 1979:215). If his and Blendon's predictions are accurate, the system as it has been pictured in this article will remain the same along with its disparities.

Returning to our discussion of urban-rural linkages in the health system, Lampton (1978:628) suggests that a central problem is how limited resources are shared between the two segments. He contends that in the tight economic situation, any shifting of resources to rural areas will cause a deterioration of the chronically limited urban resources. Yet, if the urban institutions do not support and contribute to the rural health network, their own facilities and personnel will be taxed beyond capacity. So while the urban medical profession may resist erosion of funds or time spent in rural medical training programs and rural service, the rural system will be in increasing competition for the national health care budget. An emphasis on local "self-reliance" can only be developed to a certain point. The more remote the facilities and the lower the economic levels of remote facilities, the greater will be the need for outside (i.e., municipal, provincial or central government) assistance.

RURAL HEALTH POLICY IN 1981

Fall of 1981 brought a new series of health policy statements and assertions of health accomplishments for the PRC. The Ministry of Health announced that "rural health service has been improved." Two thousand (out of 2,057) counties, 50,000 communes and "most" production brigades are now said to have a three-level health care system. Rural areas have 1.5 million Barefoot Doctors and 1.48 million doctors, nurses and pharmacists. A new policy aimed at the professionalization of BFDs has produced one-third of them having qualified for "Country doctor" certificates (to the level of assistant doctors with two to three years of training). They have obtained certification by exam, length of service of previous military service. The Ministry also released a variety of statistics (see Table 3.7) (Mainland China Press 1981).

All of these figures overwhelmingly attest to remarkable progress and impressive accomplishments. They indicate that a dedicated and innovative nation, still predominantly agricultural, still pre-industrial can make great strides in health and health care delivery. However, such numbers still can mask important geographical disparities. And, indeed, additional policy statements are revealing on the subject of disparities, if only by inference.

The Ministry of Health statement goes on to say that further decentralization of decision-making and management is to take place focusing on the provinces and the counties. The State Ministry of Health is to concentrate on policy-making and planning. Most important, particularly for the analysis presented here, is the decision with reference to payment patterns. The Ministry will encourage even greater local funding but will provide increased national financial assistance to the poorest rural sections of the country (Taylor 1981).

This new policy direction appears to recognize just precisely the rural and the urban-rural disparities that this and other research have been able to substantiate. But in our most recent (1981) observations, the Ye County health system has already been receiving substantial central government subsidy even though it has had a wealthier and successful health care system for some time. What remains is to study the impact of new policy on areas like Nong An County and those rural areas never visited to see the extent of central government aid and whether such counties are transformed from Traditional to western models in the process.

DISCUSSION

Social variables permit the prediction that national health policy is unevenly implemented throughout the People's Republic of China. The emphasis is on local initiatives, therefore, varying patterns of agricultural success and proximity to large urban centers are major correlates in how effectively policy is put into effect. It is doubtful that the PRC will be able to upgrade the system until economic conditions improve significantly, and improvement will be closely tied to the agricultural output and the success of current modernization goals which are easier set than accomplished.

There has been little examination of quality of care being delivered, and this subject certainly merits further research attention. Assuming that visitors are shown the best facilities, one can predict the quality is uneven. By western standards, old technology, the use of Traditional (and often untested) medicine and techniques, the varying educational standards for medical personnel and the obvious poverty of the health care system are bothersome. By the same token, impressive gains in health status statistics and improved health standards force us to ask just how much and what levels of equipment, personnel and facilities are actually needed to impact on health status. It has almost become a cliche to point out that sophisticated medical treatment is not a consistent correlate of the health status of a nation after certain levels in standard of living are met. It is clear from the hospital case studies presented in this paper that the Chinese are still dealing with some infectious disease problems that have all but disappeared from western nations, but their gains have been remarkable as the statistics suggest.

Mao's original health policies, which sought to emphasize rural care, may be the single policy associated with his name to be continued under the current leadership which has generally downplayed Mao's influence. The current leadership has also reached back to resurrect a pre-Communist concept that attempted to build a rural system focused around the County Health Bureaus. It may be surmised that the rural system is full of counties like Nong An, in an intermediate stage of development with a heavy Traditional medicine emphasis. The central government has now pledged itself to push them towards what Ye County has achieved with its predominant western emphasis.

Again, it is necessary to remember the lesson that policy and implementation are distinctly different. Agricultural failures may undercut resources. And one may predict severe competition for limited national resources from the urban-based physicians now studying the latest western medical techniques and technology in American, Japanese and European medical centers. They will want support for bringing these to the PRC and their values are now much more compatible with the current leadership than was true under Mao.

The most important implications of this description and discussion is that the PRC model of rural health care delivery is not able to distribute resources equitably. Its application calls for special resource support from the central government in the poorest rural areas if equity is to be achieved.

Close analysis of the PRC model increases our general understanding of processes that underlie all health care systems as they come to grips with problems of distribution of resources, equitable access, cost and quality of care and particularly with the political will and determination necessary to implement policy under formidable circumstances. A rural network of five-tiered facilities is in place in the People's Republic of China, where little existed before. This alone is impressive and merits admiration. But it is necessary to examine the realities beneath a surface description of this model of rural health care delivery to understand the problems in putting it into place and assessing its applicability to other developing nations. To laud it as a model is not enough.

NOTES

1. In the literature, one finds several terms used to describe commune-level medical facilities. They are referred to as "hospitals," "centers" and "clinics." Whether the varying terms are a reflection of arbitrary choice of words by translators or whether they have more precisely different meanings is unclear. If the latter is accurate then the terms most likely differentiate between commune facilities that have in-patient beds and those which do not.

2. There is some confusion in the literature concerning how a rural district commune hospital functions. One interpretation is that it serves the needs of several communes who do not each have their own hospital. The other interpretation is that it serves a cluster of other commune hospitals on a somewhat higher level of expertise and specialization. Clarification is needed on this point.

3. Current exchange rate is: \$1 = 1.671 Yuan; 1 Yuan = \$.60 according to the Detroit Bank-Foreign Exchange Department, May, 1982. A fen is the smallest unit of a Yuan.

TABLE 3.1
County Characteristics

	NONG AN	YE
Population	960,000	827,500
Communes	30	27
Brigades	350	1,010
BFDs/Population	1:800	1:374
Budget (Total) for whole		
Med/Health System	1,600,000 ¥	1,300,000 ¥
County Hospital		
Beds	350	186
Out-patient	800/d	560/d
Visits/Person	1=3.3	1=4.1
In-patient	9,800	7,123
Turnover	28	38.4
Occupancy	80%	86%
Herb Garden	Yes	No
County Success Rates		
Cure	86%	88.6%
Improved	11.7%	17.4%
Transferred	.5%	.4%
[Same or Worse]	[0%]	
Mortality	1.8%	4.4%*
County Staff		
Total Staff	415	213
Medical Personnel	294 (71%)	160 (75%)
Western	96	40
Traditional	9	1
Nurses	140	46
Beds/Physician	3.3	4.5
Beds/Nurse	2.5	4.0
County Salaries: Doctors and Nurses		
Highest	150 ¥	80+¥
Lowest	60 ¥	50 ¥
County: Members of CCP		
Percent Members	13% -- (Western style doctors in county)	19% -- (Only doctors in hospital, 15 of 78)
Major Health Problems: Adults		
	Bronchitis Winter) Urinary Tract Infection Arthritis GI Disorder (Summer)	Digestive Hypertension Mental Problems (Insomnia)
Major Health Problems: Children		
	Pneumonia; 2% Mortality (24/1,200 in 1978)	Pneumonia Renal Disorders GI Disorders

Source: Study Journals 1979, 1981.

TABLE 3.2
County Hospitals

	Ye 1981	Nong An 1979	Tao Yuan 1977	Heng 1977	Chang An 1977	Shunyl 1971
Population	827,500	960,000	880,000	780,000	700,000	450,000
No. Communes	27	30	60	20		19
Beds	186	350	200	145	150	155
Medical Workers	160	294	106		151	143
Doctors	41	105		83		48
5 Year	31	96		26		
3 Year	9			57		
Traditional	1	9		--		
Nurses	46	140	110	415	600	63
Out-Patients Per Day	560	880				608
In-Patients	7,123	--	4-5,000	4,000		3,474
Occupacny Rate	86%	80%*				95%
Budget	1,300,000¥	1,600,000¥	130,000¥	300,000¥	510,000¥	
Beds/1,000	.22	.36	.23	.19	.34	.21
Pop/Visit	4.1	3.0	21.9	5.2	2.0	3.2
Turnover*	38.4	.28	20-25	27.6	22.4	--
Length of Stay	8.2 days	--			15.3	
Funds/Bed	7,000¥	4,571¥	650¥	2,689¥	--	3,400¥
Funds/Person	1.57¥	1.60¥	.15¥	.50¥	--	.72¥

* Turnover Rate = In-patient Admissions/Beds

Average Length of Stay = $\frac{(360)\ (beds)}{In\text{-}patients}$ x (Occupancy)

Sources: Study Journal 1979, 1981.
       See Table 1.2 for other location references.

TABLE 3.3
Central District Hospitals

	KaiAn 1979	Chuan Shan 1977	Houshan 1979
Population	29,782	18,600	57,934
No. Communes Supported	5-6	4	90
Beds	51	20*	95
Medical Workers	43	23	13
5 Year %	9		12
3 Year %	3		24
Nurses	10		90
BFD	49		
Location	Rural	Kwelin, suburb of	Rural
Beds/1,000	1.7	1.1	1.6
Doctors/Pop.	1:2481	--	1:2317
5 Year %	75%	--	52%
3 Year %	25%	--	48%
Doctors/BFD	1:4.3	--	1:3.6
Nursery/BFD	1:5.1	--	1:3.8
Budget/BFD	1040¥	3500¥	643.7¥
BFD/Pop.	1/608	--	1/644
Budget	53,000¥	70,000¥	41,120¥
Out-patients/Day	--	108	160
In-patients	--	97	--

*Observation Only
Sources: Study Journal 1979
See Table 1.2 for other location references.

TABLE 3.4
SHIN HUA Commune--Suburban Canton: A Ten-Year Portrait

	1981	1978	1976	1974	1972	1971
General						
-Population	71,000	69,000	63,000	63,600	62,000	60,000
-Households	15,000		--	--	--	
-Brigade/Teams	20/314	20/313			21/	
-BFDs	35	35	35	25	20	20
Medical Workers	98	80	80		45	30
-Total Med						
-Total Phy	38	30				
-5 Year	5		4		7	
-3 Year	27		16		3	
-Traditional	6					
-Nurses	20				6	
-Adm/Tech/etc.	[40]				21	
-Health Aides	300+					
-BFD	138	130			36	
Out-patient	300					
-Hospital	400		300/d		300/d	
-Clinic	700		300/d		300/d	
-Total	2	1				
Health Station						
In-patient Admit	1,000/yr					
Income/Worker	831¥/yr					
Income/Capita	280¥/yr					
Staff at stat.	10+ #1					
	6-7 #2					
Budget Total	200,000¥/yr				120,000¥/yr	
-Wages, etc.	160,000¥					
-Sub-sal, equip, etc.	31,000¥					

Sources: Study Journal 1981; Sidel, New, McKinnon, Kleinman and Mechanic, Rogers (See Table 1.2).

TABLE 3.5
Four-Commune Comparison

	MALU 32,000	SHIN HUA Two Hospitals 71,000-2	5 MAY 39,000	YE 26,300
Budget Household Beds/1,000	4.0 1.06 70%+ (33)	.98 80% (44) 1:362	4.3 1:650 60	3.8 .65 1:611
Medical Workers Population 5 Year % BFD/Pop.	469 20% 1:646	1:514	1:433 900	22% 1:350
Income/Person Out-patients	Average 367 2.06 260/day 5% referral	230¥ 300 in private		200¥ 3.3
Funds/Bed/Cap.	900-1,200 1.3	5.6		5.7
Budget Infant Mortality Death Rate Financial Information	30,000-40,000* 18.2/1,000 6.3/1,000 10 fen reg/visit 2¥ year to fund total	Monthly 30 fen to Coop	2 ¥/year	151,000¥

Source: Study Journal 1979, 1981.

108

TABLE 3.6
Urban-Rural Comparisons

	Population	Hospital Beds	Beds/Pop.	Medical Workers	Med Workers/ Population
Urban					
Harbin	2.3 million	14,546	1:158	28,457	1:80
Rural					
MaLu Commune	31,000	33	1:939	66	1:469
Shin Hua Commune	35,500	44	1:806	98	1:362
Ye Commune	26,300	17	1:1547	43	1:611
5th May Commune	39,000	--	--	60	1:650

Source: Study Journals 1979, 1981.

TABLE 3.7
Health Status and Delivery System: Current Statistics

	1949	1980
Mortality Rates		
Mortality Rate	25/1,000	6.2/1,000
Infant Mortality	200/1,000	20-30/1,000 (rural) 12.8/1,000 (Peking) 12/1,000 (urban)
Life Expectancy (M&F)	35	68
Facilities & Personnel		
Hospital Beds	80,000	1.928 million
Barefoot Doctors		1.5 million
Medical Workers	5 million	2.8 million (1.48 rural)
"Health Establishments" 3,670	180,553	55,413
Commune clinics		
Medical Colleges	22,109	
Teaching Staff		30,000
Graduates	9,000 (1929-1949)	406,000 (since 1949)
National Medical Research Centers		9
Disease Patterns		
Cases of Malaria	30 million	"a few million"
Cases of Schistosomiasis	10 million	2.5 million
Smallpox		wiped out
Bubonic plague, VD, Kalazar, typhus, relapsing fever		"almost been eliminated"

Source: Mainland China Press, 30 September 1981.

Figure 3.1
Rural Health Care System

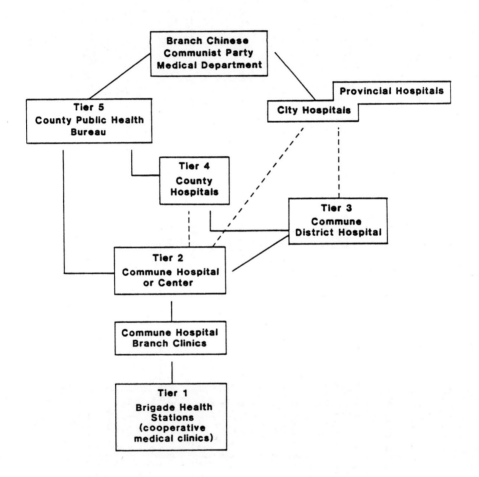

Figure 3.2
County Hospital Case Study: NONG AN

Communist Party Branch Medical Committee

County Health Bureau

NONG AN County Hospital

Departments:

Internal Medicine
Surgery
ENT
Pediatrics
Physical Therapy
Traditional Medicine
Lab/X − ray
Pharmacy
Maternity
Cardiology
Out − patient Clinics
Research
Nursing School
Training for BFD
Out − patient Health Stations 4
Herbal Garden (217 specimens)

Referral Network:

District Hospitals 9
Commune Health Centers 30
Production Brigade Clinics 350

Source: Study Journal, 1979.

112

Figure 3.3
County Hospital Case Study: YE

Communist Party Branch Medical Committee

County Health Bureau

orthopedic unit
sanitary and anti−epidemic station
drug inspection station
skin disease station
maternity and child care station

YE County Hospital

In−patient Departments:
internal medicine
surgery
physical therapy
opthamology
denistry
ob/gyn
pediatrics
pharmacy
X−ray
lab
EM

Out−patient Departments:
(established 1981, doubling the medical staff)

Referral Network:
commune district hospitals 4
commune hospitals with beds 23
production brigade clinics 1,010

Source: Study Journal, 1981.

Figure 3.4
KAIAN District Commune Hospital

District Commune Hospital

(Services KaiAn and Five Other Communes)

Departments:

laboratory
X − ray room
cardiograph room
treatment room
injection room
pharmacy
medicine production
herb garden (310 specimens)
barefoot doctor education

Referral Network:

coop medical clinics 12

Resources:

in − patient beds 51
rooms 72
staff 43
barefoot doctor 49

Source: Study Journal, 1979.

Figure 3.5
SHIN HUA People's Commune
 (Surburan Canton)

```
┌──────────────────────────────────────────────┐
│ Communist Party Branch Medical Committee       │
└──────────────────────────────────────────────┘

        ┌──────────────────────────┐
        │ County Health Bureau      │
        └──────────────────────────┘

        ┌──────────────────────────────────┐
        │ Two Commune Hospitals             │
        │                                    │
        │          Departments:              │
        │                                    │
        │       internal medicine            │
        │            X – ray                 │
        │            surgery                 │
        │           pediatrics               │
        │            ob/gyn                  │
        │              lab                   │
        │             ENT                    │
        │      traditional medicine          │
        │        no herb garden              │
        │    out – patient clinics  (2)      │
        │    (38 doctors – 20 nurses)        │
        └──────────────────────────────────┘

        ┌──────────────────────────────────┐
        │        Commune Data:               │
        │                                    │
        │      population  71,000            │
        │      households  15,000            │
        │   production brigades  20          │
        │   production teams  314            │
        │            BFD  138                │
        │       team clinics  314            │
        │      health aides  200             │
        │     medical workers  98            │
        │           beds  44                 │
        └──────────────────────────────────┘
```

Source: Study Journal, 1981.

Figure 3.6
MALU People's Commune
(Suburban Shanghai)

Commune Hospital

Departments:

ob/gyn
lab
R
BFD training
no X-ray
no surgery
no herb garden

Resources:

beds 33
medical workers 66
traditional 5
western 6
23 assistant doctors

Commune Data:

population 31,000
households 7,700
production brigades 17
health workers 54
medical coop clinics 17
54 workers
production teams 15
BFD 48
Total 3 year
some herb gardens
mostly Western medicine

Source: Study Journal, 1981.

Figure 3.7
5th MAY People's Commune
 (Suburban Shenyang)

Commune Hospital

Departments:

pharmacy
X−ray
physical therapy
surgery
EKG
out−patient (Traditional Medicine)
two internal
medicine rooms
lab
BFD education

Resources:

medical workers 60

Referral Network:

production brigades 17
production teams 86
barefoot doctors 90
medical coop clinics 17
herbal gardens

Source: Study Journals, 1979.

Figure 3.8
YE County Commune Hospital

Commune Data:

population 26,300
households 6,900
average income 218Y
(1980)   250 kg grain

Commune Hospital

Departments:

surgery
pharmacy
laboratory
denistry
maternal — child
public health
X — ray
EKG
no herb gardens

Resources:

production brigades 23
fishing brigades 3
clinics 23
BFDs 75
production teams 124
some herb gardens

Source: Study Journal 1981.

118

Figure 3.9
URBAN HEALTH CARE SYSTEM: HARBIN
(Heilungkian Province)

PROVINCIAL MEDICAL
EDUCATION
Medical College
Traditional Chinese
Medical College

PROVINCIAL-MUNICIPAL
SPECIALTY HOSPITALS
Pediatrics
Maternity
Tuberculosis
Infectious Disease
Mental Illness
Tumors
Occupational Disease

PROVINCIAL-MUNICIPAL
HOSPITALS
General
Government

HARBIN MUNICIPAL PUBLIC
HEALTH BUREAU

SEVEN MUNICIPAL DISTRICTS

PREVENTION CENTER
TB
Infectious Disease

HOSPITALS
at least one
in each district

CLINICS
Maternal
Pediatric

NEIGHBORHOOD HEALTH
CARE STATIONS

URBAN AREA   HEPATITIS   RURAL

Neighborhood Lane Health
Care Centers

Source: Study Journal 1979.

REFERENCES

Blendon, Robert J.
1979 Can China's Health Care be Transplanted Without China's Economic Problems. New England Journal of Medicine, Vol. 300, No. 26.

Chang, Tza-Kvan
1965 The Development of Hospital Services in China. Chinese Medical Journal 84:412–416. In Serve the People: Observation on Medicine in the People's Republic of China, Sidel and Sidel.

Croizier, Ralph C.
1968 Traditional Medicine in Modern China. Cambridge: Harvard University Press.
1973 Traditional Medicine as a Basis for Chinese Medical Practice. In Medicine and Public Health in the People's Republic of China. J. R. Quinn, Ed., Bethesda, Maryland. Geographic Health Studies Program, John E. Fogarty International Center for Advanced Study in the Health Care Sciences, US DHEW, Public Health Service, National Institutes of Health, DHEW Publication No. (NIH) 72–67, 3–21.

Djukanovic, V., and Mach, E. P., Eds.
1975 Alternative Approaches to Meeting Basic Health Needs in Developing Countries: A Joint UNICEF/WHO Study. Geneva: World Health Organization.

Gordon, Jeoffrey B.
1973 The Organization and Financing of Health Services. In China Medicine as We Saw It. J. R. Quinn, Ed. Bethesda, Maryland. Geographic Health Studies Program, John F. Fogarty International Center for Advanced Study in the Health Sciences, U. S. DHEW, Public Health Service, National Institute of Health, DHEW Publication No. (NIH) 75–684, 63–93.

Lampton, David M.
1974 Health, Conflict, and the Chinese Political System, Michigan Papers in Chinese Studies, No. 18. Ann Arbor: The University of Michigan Center for Chinese Studies.
1978 Development and Health Care: Is China's Medical Programme Exportable? World Development 6:621–630.

120

Mainland China Press
    1981 30 September. "Public Health Ministry Announces Achievements" Summaries of Mainland China Press. FBIS-CHI K15 China: PRC National Affairs.

Mao Tse-tung
    1965 Medical Education and Health Services, Red Medical Battle Bulletin. 18 August 1965. Translated in Survey of the China Mainland Press Supplement 198:30, 1967. Rifkin, in Medicine and Public Health in the People's Republic of China, p. 89).

Mechanic, David and Arthur Kleinman
    1978 Rural Health in the People's Republic of China Report of the Visit by the Rural Health Systems Delegation from the Committee of Scholarly Exchange with the People's Republic of China, US DHHS Public Health Service (NIH) No. 81–2124.

    1980 Ambulatory Medical Care in the People's Republic of China: An Exploratory Study. American Journal of Public Health. Vol. 40, No. 1:62–66.

New China Monthly
    1950 The Correct Direction in People's Health Work, 13, 166.

    1980 1 May, Daily Reports of Mainland China press.

    1981 15 February, New York Times

New, Peter Kong-ming
    1974 Barefoot Doctors and Health Care in the People's Republic of China. Ekistics 226:220–224.

Orleans, Leo
    1977 China's Birthrate, Deathrate, and Population Growth: Another Perspective, Congressional Research Survey Library of Congress, Washington, DC.

Rifkin, Susan B.
    1950 Peoples China: 9–11 October 1, 1950 cited in Rifkin, 1973.

    1973 Health Care for Rural Areas. In Medicine and Public Health the People's Republic of China. J. R. Quinn, Ed. Bethesda, Maryland. Geographic Health Studies Program, John E. Fogarty International Center for Advanced Study in Health Sciences, US DHEW Public Health Service, National Institutes of Health, DHEW Publication No. (NIH) 72–67, 141–152.

Seldon, Mark
1972 China Revolution and Health. Health/PRC Bulletin No. 47:16–17. In China Medicine as We Saw It, p. 72.

Sidel, Victor W. and Ruth Sidel
1973 Serve the People: Observations on Medicine in the People's Republic of China. Boston: Beacon Press.
1974 The Delivery of Medical Care in China. Scientific American 230:19–27.
1975 The Health Care Delivery System of the People's Republic of China. In Health by the People, Geneva: World Health Organization.
1977 Primary Health Care in Relation to Socio-political Structure. In Social Science and Medicine 11:415–419.
Study Journal of the UM-D/MSU Health Care Study Tour to the People's Republic of China
1979
1981
Taylor, Carl E. M.D., Dr. P.H.
1981 Summary of Trip Report. China/US Collaborative Agreement: Joint Task Force on Health Services Research. January, 1981. Johns Hopkins School of Public Health.
Tsui, Wai-ying
1979 Regionalization and Accessibility of Rural Health Services in the People's Republic of China: A Comparative Case Study of the Huancheng and Dowhan Communes. Dissertation, Chinese University of Hong Kong under supervision of Professor Rance Lee.
Wang, Chiang-wen
1978 China's Progress in Medical and Health Work. People's Republic of China Mission to the United Nations Press Release, No. 79, 12 September.
Wen, Chi-Pang and Charles W. Hays
1976 Health Care and Financing in China. Medical Care 14:241–254.

4
FAMILY PLANNING AT THE GRASS ROOTS: A
DIVERSITY OF APPROACHES

INTRODUCTION

Clearly one of the key factors in China's modernization is the success or failure of its extraordinary Family Planning Program. With one quarter of the world's population, 80 percent of whom are rural peasants, the need to control the rate of population growth is among the most urgent in the nation. With its well-known policy and programs, the People's Republic of China is attempting to create the kind of demographic transition associated with the natural dynamics of industrialization before that industrialization, and the socioeconomic conditions associated with it, take place.

All third-world countries have some fertility-limiting policy although Asia leads the current movements, being more rigorous in its family planning efforts than Africa or Latin America. This is a reflection of the enormous ecological pressures in Asia which is more densely populated than other parts of the world. In general, fertility-limiting policies range from official and unofficial promotion of outmigration to control of marriage and birth rates. The correlates of a relatively successful policy are economic development, political commitment to family planning programs and the organizational capacity to implement programs. It is most common for central economic planning units to become the source of anti-natal planning. For example, the 1953 census figures alarmed public health officials in the People's Republic of China as they saw that one of the results of the success of the Revolution was an noticeable increase in the birth rate. They went directly to the central economic planners of the country with their concerns. There remains, however, the conflict between left political ideologies which are generally pro-natal, and pragmatic considerations of enough food, enough jobs and the conditions that will promote economic growth and modernization.

In the immediate post-revolutionary period in China, an official pro-fertility attitude prevailed supported by the traditional cultural emphasis on large families with many sons. The death rate declined sharply but basically, it was not an issue that commanded official attention. Mao Tse Tung "believed that the Chinese people no matter how numerous, could construct the material basis for prosperity: 'revolution plus production' would solve all problems" (Keyfitz 1984:93). While the 1953 Census figures sounded the first alarm and stimulated concern, a strong and well-developed program did not emerge until the early 1970s with the Third Birth Planning Campaign that emphasized two-child families under the slogan: Later (marriage), Longer (time between children) and Fewer. By 1978, this approach had been transformed into the one-child campaign. In 1980, the national goal became an ultimate constant population of 1.2 billion and in December, 1982 the National People's Congress adopted a new national constitution which included an article stating that each married couple has a duty to do family planning. The PRC became the first nation in the world to make such a constitutional statement (Croll 1985).

An official Chinese description of the evolution of family planning policy delineates four periods (Qian 1984). The first period, 1949–1952, was one of "unplanned growth, a substantial drop in the mortality rate, and a rise in the birth rate of from 16/1,000 in 1949 to 20/1,000 in 1952." From 1953 to 1970, the second period began to establish policy for birth control and urban experimental programs were implemented. Studies and initial programs were implemented in the area of contraceptive production as well. The Cultural Revolution, however, set all this back. The third period, during the early 1970s was one of more rigorous implementation of a state plan for a two-child norm. The fourth and current period was launched in 1978 by the Third Plenary Session of the 11th

Party Central Committee which promulgated the one-child program.

Four primary arguments have been advanced to defend China's uniquely rigorous policy and programs to control its rate of population growth (Keyfitz 1984:40–41). The scarcity of agricultural resources has dictated strong control of food distribution through a system of rationing that emphasizes an "healthy if austere diet for all." Official sources state, however, that 10 percent of the population remains underfed. Eleven percent of the Chinese land mass, all that is arable, is under intense cultivation. Too rapid population growth would upset this tenuous situation. The modernization and economic development goals require as much capital development as possible. A lower population growth rate guarantees more capital for the modernization process. Too many young people will further exacerbate the shortage of jobs, particularly for educated urban youth and for rural youth in agricultural areas that are mechanizing. Finally, it is argued that uncontrolled population growth will create urban-rural tensions as the pressure of population movement to the cities increases.

A variety of current efforts are addressing these issues. Official encouragement of private plots for growing food to be sold on the free market (called the 'household responsibility system'), opportunities for private service enterprise and jobs, the slow-down of rural mechanization and the promotion of light industry in the countryside, the official control of population movements, and the implementation of the most vigorous family planning program known are all working to address the problems that surround population growth.

The Family Planning Program and the campaigns that implement it are a combination of educational efforts on the community and individual levels, easy access to contraceptive technologies for all married couples, a complicated array of positive and negative personal incentives and a pervasive family planning organizational structure well versed in the uses of social persuasion.

China's recent one-child family planning policy has been of great interest to visiting foreigners ever since information about it has been available. It intrigues for a variety of reasons. Because it is incarcerated in China's constitution; because it has been pursued with political rigor; because it reflects the essential need to control population in order to modernize; because it looms as a symbol of state intrusion on the most intimate decision of individual life. An opportunity to gather information on the grass roots implementation of the one-child policy presented itself during a study tour of the People's Republic of China in 1981. Many reports of the Family Planning Program have described its characteristics but until recently, few have examined the variation in its local implementation. Material systematically gathered during the 1981 study tour provides insights into the local variations that could be found in a variety of geographic locations and work settings around the country that year.

While the descriptions that follow in no way resemble formal social science research, they do provide clues as to the manner in which the family planning policy is being interpreted and put into place. The study tour visited facilities in two provinces — Shandong and Guangdong, a number of cities, and included urban, suburban and rural facilities. Shandong, where many of the rural and urban visits took place, is one of the three most densely populated provinces in China. The places visited where family planning questions were asked include rural and suburban villages (called communes in 1981), urban residential neighborhoods, two factories in towns in Shandong province, and a county health bureau in Shandong. It is possible to pair these visits to compare information gathered, particularly to contrast similar facilities and to observe the urban-rural differences. It should be noted that foreign visitors are shown what are considered "model" facilities (Study Journal 1981).

FAMILY PLANNING CONTRAST, 1981

Suburban Communes

Two suburban communes, one near Canton and one near Shanghai provided the most dramatic example of the differences the study group found. The Shin Hua Commune in suburban Canton and the MaLu Commune in suburban Shanghai took basically different approaches to implementing the family planning program. The Canton commune had some of the incentives that are among those found all over the country: people with fewer children will have more job choices; those with more than two children will not get the growing number of factory jobs available; people with more children will not get more than one or two private plots; parents must pay for abortions beyond the second child. However, the administrator of this commune of 15,000 households stated that the commune remained quite "traditional" and encouraged two children. "Two are OK," he said. The program is implemented through "general education." And of the 2,000 eligible couples, 170 have signed one-child certificates or 8.5 percent. The administrator conveyed a much more relaxed approach then was articulated in other facilities.

By contrast, MaLu, a suburban commune near Shanghai, while smaller with 7,700 households, pursued a more vigorous program with more elaborate incentives and a much higher rate of eligible couples (80 percent) having signed one-child certificates. If a couple signed the certificate, they received a twenty yuan prize and an additional four yuan a month. Their one child was guaranteed free education and two adult grain rations as well as an additional private plot. Tubal ligation incentives included one month's leave with workpoints; vasectomy gets one-half month's leave with work points. If there is a second pregnancy, no workpoints will be deducted while the woman is in the hospital. The program is clearly more elaborated and more vigorously implemented in the Shanghai suburban commune.

Urban Neighborhoods

A comparison of two urban neighborhoods, however, one in Tsing Tao and one in Shanghai, revealed very little difference. Each has a wide array of incentives, each pursues rigorous campaigns and group discussions (both at work and in the neighborhood) to persuade young couples to sign one-child certificates. The Tsing Tao neighborhood reported that 700 of 710 (98.5 percent) of eligible couples hold one-child certificates while the Shanghai neighborhood reports 94.7 percent with one-child certificates. Tsing Tao is a large city but not the size of Shanghai, one of the most populous cities in the country.

The programs and progress reported in both were similar although they are in different provinces.

Rural Brigades

Visits to two rural brigades in Shandong Province revealed the disparities found in comparing the two suburban communes near Canton and Shanghai. Dong Fang Hong Brigade, some distance from the city of Jinan, reported 90 percent of women of child-bearing age holding one-child certificates. Their incentives included a thirty-yuan prize and fifty workpoints a month for signing the certificate, free education and medical care for the one child as well as priority for land to build a house. Having a second child triggers negative incentives including no grain supply for the second child and revocation of priority for building a house although a free abortion and no loss of workpoints are also part of the incentives. One village in the Chei-Liang Brigade in Ye County, which offered 120 Yuan annual increment and an adult grain allotment for the single child, reported that only 43 percent of eligible women had signed one-child certificates. While figures for the entire brigade were not available, the contrast between the two figures suggests the disparities that may exist among villages *within* brigades.

City Factories

It was also possible to compare two factory settings in two different cities of Shandong Province. It is also the workplace, along with the neighborhood that is the focus of the family planning program. In Wai Fong, the weaving factory's employees are 60 percent women, 1,000 of whom are of child-bearing age. One hundred of these have signed a one-child certificate, or 10 percent of the eligible women. This factory offers a thirty yuan prize for signing plus a regular addition of five yuan per month. It also gives priority for new housing and priority for the single child in educational opportunity. They were contemplating allowing only daughters to inherit their father's jobs which had previously been a prerogative of sons.

The Wai Fong factory had a staff of four who worked full-time on the family planning program, yet one had a sense that the program was not pursued with particular rigor although it was not possible to ascertain why.

The Tsing Tao locomotive factory was much larger than the factory in Wai Fong. Tsing Tao is also a considerably larger city. Among its employees were 2,400 women who constituted 20 percent of the work force. This factory had a staff of four who worked full-time on family planning as well, but they carried out their work with great diligence and persistence, asking each worker to marry late (this was defined as after twenty-five) and have only one child.

The family planning workers organized small worker study groups within the factory for educational purposes. They also offered a long list of incentives and several of these were unique in terms of all the incentives the study group encountered across the country. These included 112 days of post-partum leave with pay and the possibility to stay home for three years at 70 percent of pay with a single child. There was first priority for a new or better apartment and the guarantee that an only daughter would get her father's job. We were told that "almost all" of the women had signed one-child certificates.

County Health Bureau

One final briefing on family planning took place with the Director of the Public Health Bureau of Ye County, an affluent county with a population of 827,500, twenty-seven communes and 195,000 households. This county aggressively pursues one-child certificate participation by asking couples to sign at the time of marriage. Ninety-five percent of newly married couples (probably in the last year) were said to have one-child certificates at the time of our briefing. The Director stated that "our constitution clearly states that everyone must practice family planning. It is the law . . . and the law is actively implemented in Ye County." This county officially advocates that newly married couples should live with the wife's family and the wife's family brigade is to build new housing for these couples. We were told of one brigade which "plans to build ten sets of houses for those who go to live with the wife's family."

The Director stated that as the rural economy in Ye County
grows, it will be well able to support all the elderly who need
support.

The list of incentives in the Ye County included monetary awards, guarantees of free education through the university level and free medical care as well as first priority at the
best housing. Political cadre were expected to lead the way
and set an example by being the first to sign the one-child
certificates and the county worked hard to maintain high standards of "scientific midwifery so that one child born means one
child lives."

The Range of Incentives

An overview of all the incentives offered in all locations
visited produced a remarkable array that included:

MONETARY AWARDS

Cash bonuses from 20–50 Yuan
Monthly cash of from 2–50 Yuan
Annual award of 120 Yuan

DIRECT MATERIAL AWARDS

50 additional workpoints a month
Adult grain portions for the one child
Extra private plots
Extra ration coupons for fuel and non-staple food
3-years maternity leave at 70 percent pay
Free abortion and extra workpoints on second pregnancy
Special awards of workpoints for tubal ligation and
vasectomy as well as sick leave

FUTURE PROMISES

Free education from nursery to university
First priority for new or better housing
Job guarantees for one child

Free medical care; regular check-ups for the one child
Special incentives for settling in the wife's brigade
Guarantees of care for the elderly without sons or
    daughters nearby

The precise package of incentives appeared to be related to the wealth of the unit and the determination to pursue the family planning program. But it was universal to mandate that the value of these awards be repaid if the one-child certificate was abrogated. Some units included further disincentives like no grain ration for an additional child and no extra private plots, paying for delivery of children past the first, but again, this was not mentioned everywhere.

TRANSLATION OF A ONE-CHILD CERTIFICATE

An actual one-child certificate was obtained from a commune official in suburban Canton. It was the official certificate issued by the Family Planning Office of the Guangdong provincial government. The first page of this small red booklet has spaces for the name, sex, nationality and birthdate of the child. Also the father's and mother's names, places of employment, addresses of their employers, plus a photo of the child are required. The certificate is not to be signed until the birth of the first child. A list of incentives was included. According to the translation provided by a guide and translator, the incentives printed in the booklet are as follows:

As for the one-child certificate, there are two methods: first, the child will have educational costs provided free of charge from kindergarden to senior high school; also medical service will be free until fourteen years old. Second method: urban dwellers can get five yuan per month (2.5 yuan per parent); in the countryside the child will be given some workpoints, six days of workpoints a month up to age fourteen. [Parents choose one method from the above at the time the certificate is signed]. In the commune the child will be given two pieces of land. [Parents have one per parent in addition to the child's two pieces]. As for grain, the child receives the same as for one adult. In the city, the child can get two sets of food coupons; in housing, the family with one child has the benefit of choosing the best house first. The mother will have three months of maternity leave. The parents who have one child have a priority to choose between work in the factory and agricultural work. When the family wants to build a new house, they have priority for land, raw material and labor for construction. When the child grows up, it may have priority to work in the factory. But after receiving the awards above, the mother who gives birth a second time must give the value back to the state" (One-Child Certificate 1981:2–4).

Pages five through twenty-three are left blank for the listings of medical and educational expenses, money bonuses, changes in the parents' employment and a yearly status check on the parents to guarantee they only have one child. Pages twenty-five through twenty-six contain seven further regulations: the certificate is nontransferable; it must be signed at the commune or county level; yearly updates must be kept on medical and educational expenses plus any bonuses; the choice of the award system must be noted; notification of any employment change must be made; if the certificate is lost it must be reported; and the photo must be stamped.

The wording of the document suggests that incentives would be the same (differentiating between rural and urban settings) within a province since these are so specifically spelled out in the official certificate. Yet research indicates that the incentive structure varies within work brigades in a single county and that there are differences between counties as well. This was the only certificate obtained during the study tour in 1981.

An Urban Professional Discusses Her Experience

Personal reflections on having one child were provided by the Study Tour's national guide, an urban professional woman in her early thirties. The guide Wang joined the Communist Party several years ago. Her husband is also a party member.

She signed her child certificate in 1980. She now has a daughter, about seven years old, who is a 'young pioneer' (member of an elite Communist Party young group).

Wang was one of the last people in her work unit to sign a one-child certificate. She says she was hesitant because she was afraid her daughter would become spoiled as an only child. In her work unit, all eligible couples have now signed one child certificates. There are a number of reasons why Wang decided to sign the certificate. First, by having the certificate, she receives a monthly bonus until her daughter turns fourteen. She also moved into a new apartment with two bedrooms which they got because of their one child certificate. Also having only one child gives her more freedom to pursue a career.

It appears that as a party member, it was also important that Wang set an example by signing the certificate. She denied, however, that failure to do so would have resulted in punitive action concerning her job status.

Wang's parents did not object to her signing the certificate. She indicated that they felt the choice was entirely up to her. Her in-laws, however, were more hesitant. They live in a more rural area, and still believe that 'many children bring good fortune'. Wang claims, however, that after talking with them, she and her husband were able to either change their minds or assuage their fears. In any event, the impression was that Wang and her husband are modern thinkers and that their parents have little to say over what they will eventually do. One may assume that Wang's story is one of "model" behavior.

On a number of occasions when we asked individuals their opinions of the one-child family planning program, they usually responded with some version of: "This is what the government wants." An official at the suburban Shanghai commune stated that the policy would have to be implemented until the year 2000. An official in Jinan said "The policy is only temporary."

It was clear to the study group that local areas and units are implementing the family planning policy in a diversity of ways and with varying degrees of rigor and results. Although the sample of units visited is small, hints of patterns emerge. The urban neighborhoods everywhere were similar in approach and results: high compliance rates. The two factories differed, with the one in the largest city being the most effective. Rural villages in the same county differed. And finally, suburban communes differed with the one closest to the largest city (Shanghai) showing the highest compliance. The one clear correlate appears, then, to be degree of urbanization. The higher the degree of urbanization, the greater the compliance with the one-child family norm.

The study tour only visited a handful of facilities and also was aware of problems in translation and general communication of information. However, it is possible to compare the information gathered and described here with an impressive scientific study of family planning policy implementation in four provinces, the "1982 One-per-Thousand Fertility Survey" (Freedman et al 1986).

THE ONE-PER-THOUSAND FERTILITY SURVEY

The 1982 One-per-Thousand (1/100) Fertility Survey is based on a probability survey of 815 urban and rural local units, administrative villages in the countryside (formerly called production brigades) and residence or neighborhood committees in the cities. The interview rate was an unusual 100 percent which makes the study findings commanding. These local groupings "are meaningful units of social and political organization bearing on many aspects of the lives of married couples in China . . . [reflecting] . . . on-the-spot functioning of political and economic policy." While the PRC has a powerful, centralized government working through parallel political and bureaucratic structure at all levels of governance, there is decentralization of authority. This means that national policy is influenced by local conditions and that local and individual responses are also a reflection of local conditions. Ultimately, despite relatively great centralized power, implementation of national policy is not universal.

This report of the 1/1,000 survey concentrated on rural findings in four provinces—Hebei, Henan, Liaoning and Sichuan—noting that in the provinces studied, very few urban differences could be established. "The urban neighborhoods do not differ much on the reproductive variables. This is partly because Chinese cities apparently are not very segregated by education. But further . . . the family planning program has had a much more uniform levelling effect in urban than in rural areas" (Freedman 1986:3). The 1/1,000 uncovered noteworthy rural variations within each of the four provinces among administrative villages, related to fertility rates, age of marriage, abortion ratios, proportion of first births, proportion with one-child certificates and types of contraceptives used. Some of the major findings include the following.

The percentage of the first births for administrative villages ranges from 46 percent for Henan Province to 75 percent for Hebei and 73 percent for Sichuan. Male or female sterilization as a proportion of contraception varies from 10 percent of villages to 80 percent.

There is "considerable variation" among provinces in the mix of all contraceptive methods used but greatest variation among villages within provinces. The abortion ratios, which are highest in the urban areas of each province, also vary among villages within the same province. The study notes, however, how difficult it is to judge the accuracy of all abortion reporting particularly because of the pressure on local authorities to produce high rates.

One of the most interesting findings concerns the local variations in one-child certificates. The rate for prevalence in the country as a whole, among child-bearing age couples, is 42 percent, with 78 percent being the average for the cities and 27 percent for the rural areas. In the 1/100 survey, Liaoning and Sichuan were considerably above the national rate, Hebei slightly below and Henan below. Table 4.1 presents details.

The survey also calculated a "conservative estimate" of those holding one-child certificates who go on to have more children. Almost no urban couples do this but in rural areas there is again great variation within provinces—ranging from zero to all the couples holding one-child certificates. "For China as a whole (using all women who ever had a certificate as a base) 6 percent had renounced their one-child certificate by having a second child by 1982, ranging from 0.9 percent in Beijing to 18 percent in Henan" (Freedman 1986:9). The study further reports that those who have a second child are most likely to have had a daughter first. It also notes that its own figures for those holding one-child certificates is "considerably lower" than the figures provided by the official birth planning registration system.

In the analysis of their findings, the focus was on education as a major explanatory variable. The authors of the survey conclude that the educational level of the unit as a whole has an effect on fertility beyond the education of the individual woman but that this macro-educational effect was weaker in the later years of their study. Further, a "very energetic" family planning program can "transcend overall any barriers set by low educational levels." But the program is most effective in a favorable milieu hence "it may be that the family planning program leaders realize that this is true and direct their effort more to better educated units where results will be more easily obtained" (Freedman 1986:17). There may also be a correlation between lower illiteracy and better economic conditions and lower fertility rates. At any rate, micro-educational differences in fertility are found in rural areas.

While educational levels remain a crucial explanatory variable in rural variations, the authors note that program effort and particularly the political aspects of effort remain the largely unmeasured (and unmeasurable) explanatory variable.

CONTRACEPTIVE INFORMATION

One other category of information obtained during the 1981 study tour concerned the kinds of contraceptives favored in various locations. The IUD was most mentioned everywhere, with the pill a second choice. Fifty percent of relevant women among the factory workers and urban neighborhoods used the IUD but the IUD was even more prevalent in the suburban and rural communes. These findings can be better understood by looking at some of the general literature on contraceptive development and use in the PRC. Historical material indicates considerable contraceptive research and developments for a number of decades.

Carl Djerassi, who has studied China's Family Planning Program extensively, noted in a 1973 article that since the Cultural Revolution, scientists at the Institute of Materia Medica of the Chinese Academy of Medical Sciences in Beijing and the Institute of Organic Chemistry of the Chinese Academy of Sciences in Shanghai had completed the total synthesis of the steroid contraceptive norgestrel as well as several of the naturally occurring prostaglandins. Substantial experience in the steroid chemical field already existed in the 1960s. By the 1960s, initial clinical work with a dose of norethindrone and ethinylestradiol, commonly used at that time in western countries, was performed in Shanghai. By 1969, 70–80 percent of oral contraceptive users were on a regimen of low dose combinations only considered for approval in the USA by the Food and Drug Administration in 1973.

Even more remarkable than the chemical capability and early date of clinical work with oral contraceptives is the present volume of manufacturing. It has been calculated that PRC production of oral contraceptives could suffice for 20 million women. Djerassi states that quality control is fairly primitive, however, samples collected from various cities, although of low content uniformity, were well within limits satisfactory for contraceptive efficacy.

The Chinese have pioneered a paper pill referred to as "sheet type oral birth control pill" where steroids are deposited on colored water-soluble carboxymethyl cellulose paper which is cut and perforated to give a "daily square." A "Monthly Sheet" is manufactured with twenty-two squares and is packaged automatically in cellophane envelopes.

The system for regulation of clinical testing and wide-scale distribution of chemical contraceptives is more flexible and informal than in the US. Decisions are reached through "discussions" between scientists, clinicians, and health authorities.

More recent national developments are documented in a research paper on contraceptives presented by a PRC scholar at a Swedish conference, "Research on the Regulation of Human Fertility: Needs of Developing Countries and Priorities for the Future" (Stockholm Symposium, 1983). This paper states that interuterine devices are used by 50 percent of the women who practice contraception although these devices are known to create problems of anemia by inducing increased menstrual blood loss.

The interuterine devices are most widespread in rural areas while different forms of steroid contraceptives are more popular in urban areas. What is called the "No. 1 Injectable" is increasingly rejected by urban women because it shortens menstrual periods and causes irregular bleeding. Other injectables such as megestrol acetate are increasing in popularity as they appear to give better cycle control. The well-known "Vacation pills," a long-acting oral pill containing 3 or 3.3 mg of quinestrol, is now the subject of a long-term safety study. Clinical trials of megestrol acetate-releasing vaginal rings are reported to have shown satisfactory results.

About 12 percent of women and 6 to 7 percent of men have chosen tubal ligation and vasectomy, usually after having two or more children. Studies are now underway to examine the efficacy of the chemical occlusion method and ligation with silver clips and silastic rings. This paper also reported current research on abortaficients with high efficacy and minimum side effects since "abortion forms a subsidiary but important part of the family planning program."

The Djerassi research suggests that China with a massive need for contraceptive technology, proceeded with widespread distribution while still engaged in research on side effects. These practical considerations will also offer unusual research opportunities.

The 1/100 Survey based on data analyzed in 1982 reports a much higher rate of sterilization than the Stockholm paper — 35 percent for the PRC as a whole, with more sterilization in rural than urban areas (Table 4.2). However, the survey also reports higher rates of IUD use in rural compared to urban areas with pill use more prevalent in the cities, as did the Stockholm paper. The material gathered during the 1981 Study tour on contraceptive use fits the national patterns described in this research literature.

A CASE STUDY IN FAMILY PLANNING PERSUASION

While the 1981 Study Tour did not have the opportunity to see any of the small family planning study groups in action, one study in the literature does provide a glimpse of this process.

A community study of a production brigade in Guangdong Province includes a detailed description of how birth control work is carried out in small discussion groups (Mosher 1982). While there is no claim that this description is typical, it does provide some insight into the nature of this work.

In January 1979 after the Guangdong Provincial Revolutionary Committee issued a directive calling for no more than two-child families, the party committees of various brigades were to decide whether to pursue the family planning program through household visits or group meetings. The brigade studied chose the later and included the seventy-four couples identified in a survey of the brigade's 10,000 families who did not conform to the two-child norm and other guidelines. Meetings ran from 8 am to 5 pm everyday and were patterned after the well-known "small group discussion" which has been a regular feature of Chinese life for disseminating central policy on the lowest local level.

The atmosphere of the meetings is one of open exchange rather than intimidation. Discussion focused on the consequences of birth control for the nation as a whole, for the brigade and for the individual family and woman. The women were grouped according to the number and sex of the children already in the family, along with two or three women who were cadre (political leaders). Attendance was mandatory at these daily discussions which, in the brigade studied, went on for five months. The emphasis was on persuasion but social pressure and economic sanctions made it difficult to hold out as there was a stress on the rewards of accepting contraception.

Research found that the dominant and over-riding issue was the sex of the children the women already had. Although the women understood that the limited land of the brigade could support only a certain number of people,

. . . women in this brigade customarily calculated their fertility in terms of boys, and when they agreed that two children would be enough, it was boy children that they had in mind. Girls literally don't count. Left alone, the village women would continue to bear children until they reach their desired number of boys. . . . The old tradition of emphasis on boys was extremely difficult to overcome and the emotions connected to that tradition was expressed succinctly by one of the woman. 'Women want a man-child . . . because without one you will be poor and picked on in your old age. Families with only girls have little voice in village affairs. Everyone knows that the girls sooner or later will marry out. A son will stay by your side until you pass away . . . a person without a son has nothing to lean on in old age' (Mosher 1982:359).

Despite the fact that one of the economic sanctions imposed during this brigade's discussion sessions was loss of workpoints, sixty-four of the original seventy-four continued to refuse any form of contraception. Everyone of these women either had no sons or only one son. So the old tradition continues to be a powerful one.

While it can be assumed that a wide range of educational and persuasion techniques are used throughout the 2,000,000 rural villages of the PRC, and that many do not require mandatory attendance or loss of workpoints, this one example appears to highlight the major obstacle to acceptance of a one-child family planning model.

A more recent analysis corroborates this case study. Writing about the one-child policy, Davin (1985:38) states:

Enormous pressure is exerted on peasant couples to restrict their families to one . . . This means that 50 percent of couples are being asked to face old age without a male heir and to accept that their family line will end in their generation, while all families are required to curtail their future supply of labour.

Davin continues by asserting that

The enormous intrusiveness of family planning work is well documented. The careful records enable the village family planning worker to identify her 'targets' precisely. Unmarried young people are persuaded to postpone marriage, childless couples are visited and urged to 'await their turn' to try for a pregnancy, and those who already have a child are asked to practice contraception or accept sterilization. Sterilization is the solution urged on all couples with more than one child (Davin 1985:45).

It should be noted that the government has stated firmly that "by pursuing its family planning programme, China has always followed the principle of voluntary participation under state guidance and opposed all coercive means in the work of family planning" (Beijing Review 1985:8).

SUMMARY

The number of obstacles to implementing the one-child family planning policy in the People's Republic of China are overwhelming. A recital of these obstacles makes the impressive gains of the program all the more remarkable. Mitigating against implementation are the strong traditional value placed on sons and on large families with many sons, the eldest of whom has traditionally taken care of the elderly parents. Of a more contemporary nature is the problem generated by current agricultural policy emphasizing and encouraging private plots in the countryside. The more hands, the more successful the private plots and more hands suggest larger families. These two factors alone could help explain the diversity of rural response to the one-child policy. In some villages, political cadre and family planning workers are not able to overcome the resistance offered by individual families or groups of families. Political cadre and family planning workers can only press so hard where there is strong resistance. If they push too hard against strong rural norms, they risk losing their general status and effectiveness.

Indeed, there is a recent report (Greenhaigh 1986) that there may be a limited relaxation of the one-child policy which now permits a second child for those signing certificates, but only under a restricted number of conditions. Such a concession may well be a response (at least temporarily) to the persistence of various forms of resistance.

Nonetheless, it is clear that the Family Planning Program in the PRC has been remarkably if not perfectly successful. Birth and death rate figures from a variety of sources reveal the following:

Birth Rate Decline

Year	Birth Rate
1949	35/1,000
1955–1959	25/1,000
1965–1969	44/1,000
1980	18/1,000
1982	20/1,000
1985	19/1,000

Death Rate Decline

Year	Death Rate
1949	20/1,000
1980	6/1,000

Sources: Keyfitz, 1984, p. 42.
Population Reference Bureau, 1986.

The rise in the birth rate in 1982 to 20/1,000 has been interpreted as a reflection in the decrease in death rate and in "demographic momentum" (the delayed effect of an early period of rapid population growth producing more young people of marriageable age). Therefore, the population continues to increase while fertility declines. However, the Population Reference Bureau, a private Washington DC population study group reports in 1985 that China's birthrate is down to 19 per 1,000. This has influenced the world's decline in birthrate to 27 per 1,000 people (Schmid 1985).

The choices for the PRC are not enviable ones. A faster drop in the birth rate will reduce pressure on resources but too fast a drop will require enormous social pressure and discipline and will produce an unfavorable age distribution in future years with too few workers supporting too large an elderly population. Table 4.3 suggests what this ratio might look like in the Shanghai figures. A slower decline will require less social pressure, a better age distribution but leave fewer resources available for the modernization effort (Keyfitz, 1984).

These dilemmas certainly make the descriptions of social pressure more understandable. Clearly the goal is to make national necessity and individual choice the same, an enormously difficult task. The evidence of local variation in implementation of the one-child norm is perhaps most remarkable because it is not even more widespread. China is engaged in one of the most extraordinary family planning efforts in the history of the world, one that has wide implications for the world's population and one that the world will watch closely for decades to come.

TABLE 4.1
Percentage Distribution of Production Brigades, Urban Neighborhoods, and All Local Units on Percentage of Eligible Women Holding a One-Child Certificate, 1 July 1982

% of Women with one-child cert.	Rural Production Brigades				Urban Neighborhoods				All Local Areas			
	Hebel	Henan	Liaoning	Sichuan	Hebel	Henan	Liaoning	Sichuan	Hebel	Henan	Liaoning	Sichuan
0-9	34.0	55.3	0.0	17.9	0.0	0.0	0.0	0.0	32.1	52.0	0.0	16.5
10-19	20.0	12.8	6.3	5.1	0.0	0.0	0.0	0.0	18.9	12.0	4.5	4.7
20-29	10.0	4.3	0.0	20.5	0.0	0.0	0.0	0.0	9.4	4.0	0.0	18.8
30-39	8.0	12.8	25.0	7.7	33.3	0.0	0.0	0.0	9.4	12.0	18.2	7.1
40-49	6.0	2.1	18.8	10.3	0.0	33.3	0.0	0.0	5.7	2.0	13.6	9.4
50-59	8.0	6.4	12.5	12.8	0.0	0.0	16.6	0.0	7.5	8.0	9.1	11.8
60-69	4.0	2.1	6.3	7.7	0.0	0.0	0.0	0.0	3.8	2.0	9.1	7.1
70-79	8.0	2.1	6.3	1.3	0.0	0.0	0.0	14.3	7.5	2.0	4.5	2.4
80-89	2.0	2.1	12.5	5.1	0.0	33.3	0.0	14.3	1.9	4.0	9.1	5.9
90-100	0.0	0.0	12.5	11.5	66.6	33.3	83.3	71.4	3.8	2.0	31.8	16.5
TOTAL %	100.0	100.0	100.0	100.0	100.0	100.0	100.0	100.0	100.0	100.0	100.0	100.0
No. of Units	50	47	16	78	3	3	6	7	53	50	22	85
Percent for Province	32	18	54	50	72	74	96	93	38	24	76	58

Source: Freedman et al, 1986.

TABLE 4.2
Percentage Distribution of Contraceptive Methods by Current Users,
July 1982, for Four Provinces

Methods	Rural Production Bridgades				Urban Neighborhoods				All Local Areas				China
	Hebel	Henan	Liaoning	Sichuan	Hebel	Henan	Liaoning	Sichuan	Hebel	Henan	Liaoning	Sichuan	
Tubal ligation	12	35	38	10	9	22	13	20	12	34	29	11	25
Vasectomy	1	7	1	41	2	1	1	13	1	6	1	38	10
IUD	69	55	52	43	34	52	54	36	66	55	53	42	50
Pill	11	1	6	2	33	18	16	11	13	3	9	3	9
Other	7	2	3	4	22	8	16	20	8	2	8	6	6
TOTAL %	100	100	100	100	100	100	100	100	100	100	100	100	100
Total No.	6,259	7,865	3,384	11,685	667	775	1,804	1,684	6,926	8,640	5,188	13,369	120,516

Source: Freedman et al, 1986.

TABLE 4.3
Median Age and Old-Young Ratio in Various Provinces, Municipalities and Autonomous Regions

	Median Age	% 65 Years and Older	% 14 Years and Younger	Old-Young Ratio %
National Average	22.91	4.91	33.60	14.61
1. Shanghai	29.28	7.37	18.10	40.75
2. Beijing	27.19	5.64	22.12	25.49
3. Tianjin	26.60	5.54	24.24	22.84
4. Jiangsu	25.54	5.54	28.99	19.10
5. Hebei	24.72	5.66	30.78	18.39
6. Zhejiang	24.69	5.77	29.33	19.68
7. Liaoning	24.58	4.80	28.78	16.69
8. Shandong	24.56	5.63	31.02	18.16
9. Sichuan	23.41	4.67	34.42	13.58
10. Hubei	23.02	4.99	32.76	15.23
11. Shanxi	22.99	4.99	33.31	14.97
12. Shaanxi	22.89	4.58	33.09	13.83
13. Guangdong	22.54	5.44	33.87	16.06
14. Hunan	22.48	4.97	33.92	14.66
15. Jilin	22.33	3.97	33.18	11.96
16. Henan	22.27	5.23	34.92	14.97
17. Heilong-jiang	21.58	3.42	34.83	9.83
18. Tibet	21.45	4.64	36.98	12.54
19. Inner Mongolia	21.19	3.61	35.41	10.19
20. Fujian	20.68	4.34	36.53	11.89
21. Anhui	20.18	4.08	36.15	11.30
22. Gansu	20.13	3.48	36.36	9.57
23. Guangxi	20.01	5.11	37.39	13.68
24. Jiangxi	19.67	4.51	38.90	11.60
25. Xinjiang	19.48	3.73	39.72	9.39
26. Yunnan	19.39	4.51	39.17	11.52
27. Guizhou	18.76	4.68	40.88	11.45
28. Qinghai	18.42	2.71	40.78	6.64
29. Ningxia	18.32	3.25	41.44	7.84

Note: Statistics are from a 10 percent sample survey.
Source: Beijing Review, 1984.

REFERENCES

Beijing Review
1984 "Third National Census: Age Distribution of China's Population." Vol. 27, No. 2, 9 January, pp. 20–22.

Beijing Review
1985 "China Seeks Mild Growth in 1986–1990." Vol. 28, No. 40, 1 October, pp. 6–8.

Croll, E., Davin, D., & Kone, P., (Eds.)
1985 China's One-Child Family Policy. New York: St. Martin's Press.

Davin, Delia
1985 "The Single-Child Family Policy in the Countryside," in China's One-Child Family Policy, Elisabeth Croll, Delia Davin, and Penny Kaire, eds., pp. 37–82. Macmillan.

Djerassi, Carl
1973 Steroid Contraceptives in the People's Republic of China, New England Journal of Medicine. Vol. 289, No. 10, 6 September, pp. 533–535.

Freedman, Ronald, Xiao, Zhenyu, Li, Bohua, & Levely, William.
1986 "Local Variations in Reproductive Behavior in the People's Republic of China, 1973–1982." Revision of a paper presented at the meetings of the Population Association of America, San Francisco, 2 April.

Greenhaigh, Susan
1986 "Shifts in China's Population Policy 1984–1986: Views from the Central, Provincial and Local Levels." Population and Development Review, Vol. 12, pp. 491–515.

Keyfitz, Nathan
1984 "The Population of China." Scientific American, February, Vol. 250, No. 2, pp. 38–47.

Mosher, Stephen W.
1982 "Birth Control: A View from a Chinese Village." Asian Survey, Vol. XXII, No. 4, April, pp. 356–367.

One-Child Certificate
1981 "One-Child Certificate." Family Planning Office, Guandong Province.

148

Qian Xinzhong
1984 "Evolution of China's Population Policy." Beijing Review, Vol. 27, No. 3, 16 January, pp. 17–19.

Schmid, Randolph
1985 "Chinese Head a Decline in the World's Birthrate." Detroit Free Press, 8 April, p. 13H.

Stockholm Symposium
1983 "Research on the Regulation of Human Fertility: Needs of Developing Countries and Priorities for the Future." 7–9 February, Stockholm, Sweden: Karolinska Institutet and the University of Uppsala. Lei Hai-Peng, "Contraceptive Methods Used in the PRC."

Study Journals
1979, 1981 Journal of The University of Michigan-Dearborn and Michigan State University Study Tour on Health Care in the People's Republic of China. Unpublished manuscripts available from the author upon request and deposited in the Study Tour Journal Collection, The University of Michigan.

5
FROM HERBAL GARDEN TO ASSEMBLY LINE: THE TRANSFORMATION OF A TRADITION

It was unusual to be able to visit a distant rural area in the People's Republic of China at least for visitors at the end of the 1970s and early 1980s. Therefore, our visit to Nong An County in 1979 which had not had foreign visitors since World War II provided a unique opportunity for comparisons with other rural and well-developed county health facilities, particularly with reference to use of Traditional medicine (Study Journal 1979).

CONTRASTING LEVELS OF USE

County Hospitals

Nong An County Hospital, serving a county population of 960,000, had 350 beds, and a staff of 105 doctors of various degrees of education. Nine percent of these were Traditional doctors. The hospital courtyard (and beyond) was prominently occupied by a three-mos herbal garden that contained 217 different medicinal plants. All the medical staff took turns tending the garden which was under the direction of an older Traditional doctor. The hospital had extensive facilities for drying and storing the herbs, and medicine-producing equipment as well.

The hospital director stated, with some emphasis, that the integration policy is taken "very seriously" at this hospital.

The hospital has organized study groups for western-style doctors from the communes to "cultivate their minds, to learn Chinese medicine." Acupuncture is used to treat appendicitis, gall stones, ectopic pregnancies, brain tumors, and infant pneumonia, and used as an anesthetic for thyroidectomies and difficult labor and delivery. The hospital claims a general 90 percent success rate in the use of Traditional approaches. It has completed a study of 296 cases of appendicitis. Of these, 187 were treated by operation, spent 11.8 days recovering and cost thirty yuan per person. By contrast, 109 cases were treated by Traditional methods, spending an average of 5.1 days in the hospital and cost five yuan per person. "So," the director concluded, "Traditional medicine is cheaper and quicker."

In contrast was the stance and practice of another county hospital in a more affluent area serving a similar size population of 827,500. This was Ye County (County) Hospital in Shandong Province (Study Journal 1981). Ye County is a World Health Organization model demonstration center, used to educate other health workers from around the PRC and other Third World countries. Like more health facilities in wealthier areas of the country, it did lower levels of medical work, but with more resources. It had only one Traditional doctor (this constituted 3 percent of all its staff doctors) who had some western-style training as well. He had his own out-patient acupuncture clinic and a small in-patient ward as well. However, the hospital has no herb garden, used western medicine for all acute conditions, and relatively little Traditional medicine.

Commune Hospitals

This same sort of contrast was observed, in 1979 and 1981, between suburban commune hospitals and distant rural commune hospitals. Ye Hsein People's Commune Hospital in Shandong Province and MaLu Commune Hospital near Shanghai had 4 or 5 percent of their staff who were Traditional practitioners, neither had its own herbal garden, and neither produced its own herbal medicine. MaLu reported that 20 percent of its pharmacy budget was spent on purchasing herbs;

Ye Hsein said 6 percent of its budget, and, although both said they used a combination of treatments for their patients, treatment and diagnosis were based on western medicine (Study Journal 1981).

By contract, KaiAn Commune Hospital in Nong An County, a poorer more distant area, put a heavy emphasis on Traditional medicine. It had a large herbal garden, larger than its county referral hospital at Nong An. It grew 310 varieties of medical plants, some transplanted from southern provinces, some transplanted from the wilds. It stored herbs and made extensive use of its own medicines. The garden was tended by an elderly herbalist who had learned his trade beginning as an apprentice of 10. Its staff was 10 percent traditional in basic training and the hospital also made considerable use of combined western and Traditional treatment.

These are, of course, only a very small number of instances, but they do suggest the strong economic correlates of Traditional medicine use. Where there is choice in the more urbanized and wealthier facilities, they move towards western medicines and treatments.

Traditional Hospitals and Medical Schools

Perhaps more telling is what goes on in the Traditional medical colleges of the country. There was the opportunity to visit Harbin's Learning Institute of Traditional Chinese Medicine, in 1979, and the well-known Lung Hua Traditional Hospital and Medical College, Shanghai, in 1981. Both are teaching medical students and treating in- and out-patients in 350 and 400 bed hospitals.

The majority of doctors in each hospital are traditionally trained. However, the chief medical directors and a number of chiefs of service were originally western-style trained, and after a number of years of clinical experience then took two or three-year courses in Traditional medicine. Patients in these teaching hospitals are treated with a combination of Traditional and western approaches. Thirty percent of the pharmacy at Lung Hua was of western pharmaceuticals. While many of the patients have chronic diseases, a wide variety of conditions are treated. Mentioned in the two facilities were acute appendicitis, chronic bronchitis, coronary valve disease, arterial disease, cirrhosis of the liver, tumors, cancer, other heart and circulatory diseases, gall stones, rheumatic arthritis, diabetes, chronic headache. In Harbin, observations were made of tooth extraction by acupressure in the dental clinic, and tonsils removed by cauterization.

The students in both schools have to pass a standardized national examination for admission to both Traditional and western-style medical schools. The exam includes chemistry, math, physics, political science, and the Chinese language. The programs are from four to five years. In Harbin, there was an opportunity to visit the herbal teaching room. Some 1,100 specimens from plants and animals were displayed. These had been collected by students and faculty of the college during expeditions to nearby mountains. Students were taught to identify the plants and which parts were medically useful. A special specimen table contained jars of wild ginsing, thirteen- and seventeen-years old, richer in quality than cultivated ginsing. There were powdered parts of deer antler and bones, used like vitamins for "strengthening people"; the viscera of female deer for gynecological disease; leopard bone for rheumatoid arthritis; and seahorse to improve kidney and liver function.

At both college hospitals, western diagnoses and treatment were used along with Traditional techniques. Both had western-style diagnostic equipment, like X-rays and laboratory equipment. Lung Hua's assistant director stated that the emphasis was on western approaches for in-patients and Traditional approaches for out-patients. They regularly received transfer patients from western hospitals (typically chronically ill patients), but never, we were told, transferred patients out. In both places, the typical patient was over fifty-years old.

At the Harbin Learning Institute of Traditional Chinese Medicine, there was an opportunity to talk at length with one of the elderly Traditional doctors who got his training as an apprentice to a Master. His observations were telling. "The integration of Traditional medicine with western medicine is better than treatment with Traditional medicine alone," he said. Western techniques enhanced Traditional approaches. He cited, as examples, using herbal medicines to shrink and pass gall stones but X-ray of the gall bladder for initial assessment. Another example was combining Traditional massage with painkillers. He was pleased that the students at that college studied physiological anatomy, X-ray diagnosis, pharmacological chemistry, and western-style diagnosis along with their Traditional studies.

He described particular cases where Traditional medicine cured when western medicine could not and spoke about the older people of the country who preferred Traditional medicine because it was "their own." He also described folk medicine practices still popular and useful among the farmers. From his point of view, the biggest obstacle to "true integration" was the fact that few western doctors really understood or could practice Traditional medicine very well.

In the Traditional doctor's wide-ranging remarks can be found the realities of Traditional medicine in the People's Republic of China today. It is slowly modernization and westernization.

Other hospitals and facilities like those we visited have also been described in official Chinese publications. Li Shezhen Hospital of Chinese Medicine in Qizhou, a small town in Hubei Province has been described as a model Traditional hospital (Beijing Review 1985). Named for the 16th Century Chinese medical expert, Li Shizen, it has 180 beds, a staff of 150, and combines Traditional and western approaches. It has modern equipment like an X-ray machine, electrocardiogram, and liver monitoring devices. It also has its own pharmacy factory which produces two kinds of prepared Traditional medicines and medical liquor used to treat rheumatism, based on Li's original prescriptions. Agricultural conditions in the general area are considered excellent for growing herbs and there are thirty-six medicinal herb farms in the county. Peasants also do well with private herb plots. Officials of the County's Herbal Medicines Department reported, in 1983, that the County Bureau of Public Health purchased 38,220 Kg. of medicinal herbs of which one-fifth were grown on private plots.

CASE STUDY: HERBAL MEDICINE AND APPEN-DICITIS[1]

Many settings, both rural and urban, mentioned the extensive use of herbal preparation to treat appendicitis. One member of the 1981 study tour made a careful study of the approaches used and this provides an interesting case study of one application of Traditional medicine in the PRC.

According to the Chinese Institute for Acute Abdominal Diseases appendicitis is diagnosed with both modern techniques and the Traditional methods of inspection, smelling, questioning and pulse examination. The treatment itself is based on three procedures: evacuation of the intestine, introduction of antibacterial agents, and promotion of circulation to the damaged organ (Lasagna 1975).[2]

In a ten-year study 1,130 out of 2,000 appendicitis patients were cured by herbal medicine with a mortality rate of only 0.17 percent (Institute for Acute Abdominal Disease 1978). Some 20,000 appendicitis cases have been treated non-surgically since the Cultural Revolution with a 90 percent cure rate and only 30 percent of all appendicitis cases ever undergo appendectomies (National Academy of Science 1975). There is a problem with these statistics of successful herbally treated appendicitis cases, however. There is no proof that the appendix was ever actually inflamed. Appendicitis is notoriously tricky to diagnose and at one point in America so many noninflammed appendixes were being removed that the American Medical Association set up an investigative board to review doctors with too many misdiagnosed cases of appendicitis.

The literature provides nine different herbal prescriptions for treatment of appendicitis (see Table 5.2). All nine contain an herbal laxative; eight have herbs that are used as antibacterials; seven contain plants to increase circulation. There are also five prescriptions that contain painkillers and three have herbs that control vomiting. Most of the prescriptions also contain several herbs whose purpose is not determined. Several of the herbs, such as *Rheum officinale* (rhubarb) and *Loniecere japonica* (honeysuckle) were used in multiple prescriptions.

There appears to be little Chinese research on the active components of herbs. However, there are several foreign studies on herbs and the results of these are useful. Three herbs which are used frequently — *Rheum officinale, Paeonae lactiflora,* and *Paeonae moutan* (peonies) — are significant because they contain an active component capable of producing one or more of the three alleged effects of the Chinese treatment. *Rheum officinale* contains five different anthraquinones (Shibata 1979). These increase conolic peristalsis without affecting the movements of the stomach or duodenum (Donghai 1980). Thus, rhubarb acts as a laxative and additional research indicates that it might have antibacteria effects (National Academy of Science 1975). *Paeonae moutan* contains paeonol which acts as a sedative, antipyretic, and analgesic (Shibata 1979).

Appendicitis is an ailment often treated by Barefoot Doctors with only the more serious cases being referred up to higher level facilities. This fact was discovered at an interview with a Barefoot Doctor from Ye county and at a number of facilities during the 1981 Study Tour. The Ye county Barefoot Doctor's abilities were proved to be neither unusually competent or ambitious by an interview with two suburban Shanghai Barefoot Doctors, both of whom were able to treat appendicitis. They used a combination of western antibiotics and Chinese herbs which consisted of an external plaster of garlic and mirabilite and a potable decoction.

The prescription given by one of the Shanghai Barefoot Doctors is different from those given in the literature although it contains several herbs found in the literature prescriptions. Two of the herbs, *Taraxacum officinale* and *Glycyrrhize uralensis* (licorice), have active components that have been shown to be anti-inflammatory agents. Another herb, *Loniecere japonica,* has been tested in laboratory animals. So one could say there was a "western basis" for this prescription. But the two herbs on which the most research has been done are both anti-inflammatories used in conjunction with antibiotics which seems redundant. The use of the garlic-salt plaster has no scientific basis. Grass root level treatment of appendicitis has some scientific foundation, but it still uses substances whose efficacy is not proven.

In secondary facilities such as factory and commune hospitals both herbal treatment and surgery is used. Appendectomies are performed only on serious cases, but there is a vagueness to the term "serious" that needs to be clarified. In two of the hospitals visited, the two main herbs used in non-operative treatment were *Rheum officinale* and *Paeonae moutan*, both of which have a great deal of research supporting their efficacy. These were also used in conjunction with western antibiotics. A factory hospital in TsingTao also used *Rheum officinale* as a main herb and supplemented it with acupuncture for pain and inflammation.

Treatment in secondary facilities appears to be more acceptable by western standards than treatment at the brigade level. Herbs used are more firmly entrenched in western-style proof and there is the western back-up, surgery, available. As a sidenote, there was the opportunity to interview a man who had had to utilize this back-up. Sometime in the 1950s he had been treated herbally for appendicitis when his appendix ruptured and he underwent surgery. Since that time he had another operation and was in acupuncture therapy, both of which were attempts to correct intestinal adhesions resulting from the rupture.

Information was gathered on the treatment of appendicitis in tertiary facilities at the Shanghai Municipal Traditional Hospital. Cases of appendicitis were to be found only in the surgery department. From this one can induce that the major method of treatment of appendicitis here is by appendectomy, a purely western solution.

An interesting facet of herbal treatment of appendicitis is the existence of an over-the-counter medicine. These ready-made pills are available in most pharmacies and must be fairly widely used because the two pharmacies at which they were requested carried them. These pills are for chronic appendicitis only and a doctor at the TsingTao workers' sanatorium said that acute cases required surgery. This raises the interesting possibility that all the herbal remedies may have been for chronic appendicitis which would not be surgically treated even in America.

This small case study provides a patchwork of information that does not paint a clear-cut picture. Much more research would be needed to differentiate when it is appropriate to treat with pharmaceutical agents (herbal or otherwise) and when surgery is required. Apparently, the Chinese are having considerable success with herbal approaches.

ASSEMBLY-LINE TRADITIONAL MEDICINES

An altogether different facet of Traditional medicine is found in special mechanized urban factories. The Shanghai Chinese Medicine Factory #1 offers an important clue to the transformation of Chinese Traditional medicine today (Study Journal 1981). Established in 1958, it is an amalgamation of several old and famous herbal workshops from the local area, brought together to be modernized. It began with 300 workers and now employs 800 in a factory of 20,000 square meters that is still adding sections to its spacious enclosed compound. It produces, on semi-automated assembly lines, 280 different Traditional prescriptions in a variety of pills, powders, pastes, pellets, ointments, and liquids. These recipes were chosen as the most popular and efficacious from among the hundreds brought by the various workshops that came together.

The director began his career as a thirteen-year-old apprentice to an old herbalist and got "practical" training, by learning on the job. One Traditional doctor and three western-style doctors are on the staff along with an engineer who is a medical college graduate, a college-trained engineer, as well as laboratory technicians who have college training. The plant manager has a background similar to the directors as do a number of other staff members. The factory contains several different buildings including a separate mixing building which stored raw materials on its second floor. These were sent by conveyor to crushing devices on the ground floor. Seven or eight different refining apparatus based on different techniques were in use as well as a sorting machine with water and organic solvent. Vats of liquid suspensions waited to be refined.

Quality assurance techniques varied. The director stated that thousands of years of use had established general efficacy. New medicines usually undergo three years of study on animals first, then humans. The factory does some of this research, but the bulk is carried out at medical colleges and the Academy of Traditional Medicine in Shanghai. The factory director could not recall many examples of drugs being taken off the market, only new mixtures causing the gradual demise of old ones. If well prepared, these medical preparations have a shelf life of two to three years.

Medicines are manufactured according to market requirements and have to be approved by the Shanghai Health Bureau. The factory concentrates on production of one kind of medicine in three-month cycles. Every year or two, it introduces a new product; at the time of the 1981 visit, one was under study for cardiovascular disease. A great deal of effort was going into cancer research to find a Traditional medicine that might be useful.

From the staffs' point of view, their standardization of medicines and injections represented a "great improvement from the originals" and that it was "good to move towards modernization." "We can stick to Chinese medicine, but make the methods (of production) more scientific. With the scientific way, they are more effective and the population thinks they are more effective. An old saying about Traditional medicine is still this: 'Once you look at it, you like it'." Overall, the staff of Shanghai Medicine Factory #1 felt that the great advantage of Traditional medicines was that they produced fewer side effects. They were particularly proud of the national award they had received recently for the quality of their cough medicine.

The medicine produced at Shanghai Medicine Factory #1 can be found in pharmacies in Shanghai and other large cities in China as well as in Chinatowns all over the world, including the USA. In the People's Republic of China, consumers can walk into such shops, describe their symptoms and problems and purchase medicines without a prescription. This includes both Traditional and western medicine.

While in TsingTao, it was possible to visit an herbal supply station, factory and pharmacy, and talk to members of the station's staff. The herb supply station is owned by the State and gets an annual budget of one million Yuan. The supply station has four sources of herbs: its own two-hectare plot of land just outside the city where eleven different herbs are cultivated; gardens from elsewhere in the county from which herbs in bulk are purchased; wild herbs which it gathers from around the county; and purchases made from other provinces. From this raw material, two forms of Traditional medicine are produced, the raw materials from which Traditional prescriptions are concocted and the pre-prepared medicines of the kind seen in Shanghai Traditional Medicine Factory #1.

These products are sold directly to all the drug stores in seven adjoining counties, including the thirty drug stores in TsingTao, to hospitals and small clinics in these counties which take 70 to 80 percent of the supply station's stock, and directly to the public. The supply station is serving a total population of seven million people through its own pharmacy.

The history of some of the Traditional pharmacies in the PRC is impressive. The Tongrentang Pharmacy of Beijing celebrated its 315th anniversary in February, 1985 (Beijing Review 1985). This pharmacy was founded in 1669 and became the exclusive supplier to the royal court in 1723. It produced prescriptions by court doctors as well as hundreds of secret ancient and folk recipes. Particularly reknown were its Bezoar Antifebrile Pill for fever and delirium, the white Phoenix Pill for menstrual problems and the Bezoar Chest Pill for coma induced by high fever. The Tongrentang Pharmacy consists of two drug processing workshops, a division producing medicinal liquor and a staff of 2,000. It is the largest producer of medicinal items for export.

All of the facilities described here are now under more rigorous state regulations. In 1983, a Pharmacy Reform Law was passed which imposed new standardization and quality control in the production of Traditional pharmaceuticals.

TRADITIONAL MEDICINE AS AN EXPORT ITEM

Traditional medicines are among the many items exported by the PRC. The People's Republic of China has increased its general export trade dramatically, with a twenty-fold jump between 1957 and 1980. This includes the export of herbal medicines. A *Daily Report* (1982) article notes that the State's purchases of herbal medicines increased 3.2 times between 1957 and 1980 and patent medicines increased eleven times. The US government reports that the PRC exported $198 million worth of medicines in 1982, and that this was 8 percent of its total export.

Additional data from other sources helps develop a picture of herbal medicines as an important export item for China. For example, it is possible to document that the export value of agricultural primary products (of which herbal medicines are one example) have increased dramatically.

The Direction of Trade Annual (1985) notes the value of export of primary agricultural commodities. In 1966 it was $919 million in USA dollars; in 1976 $2,053.9; in 1982 $3,169.1.

It is also possible to establish which countries are major trading partners for China, although we do not know the rate at which these countries buy herbal medicines. In 1984 China sold $10,407 million of herbs to industrial countries. Its sales of herbs to developing countries totalled $13,159 million to Africa, $9,347 million to Asia, $6,586 million to Hong Kong and $70 million to Indonesia.

Finally, Table 5.2 provides some data on the export of Traditional medicines, 1982–1985.

While it is not clear why the tonnage has fluctuated (perhaps crop failure), what is clear is that Traditional medicines are used both for internal populations as well as for export and remain an important trade item. It should also be noted that herbal medicine products are a very old export item for China. There is documentation, for example, that during the Song Dynasty from the Tenth to the Thirteenth Century, some fifty-eight kinds of Traditional medicines were shipped abroad (Beijing Review 1980).

A recently published, comprehensive British study of Traditional medicine makes this corroborating statement:

Traditional and modern pharmaceuticals are among the top fifty of China's exports. One market is the large 'overseas' Chinese population. Another is Third World countries like Algeria and Ethiopia where Chinese health teams have worked. The manufacture of Traditional products requires less capital investment than Western medicine, even if modern technology is

TABLE 5.1
Exports of Traditional Medicines

	1982	1983	1984	1985
Crude Drug Materials	18,419	21,315	19,595	16,271
Patent Medicines	6,312	6,312	5,777	6,048
	1980	1982	1984	
Crude Drug Materials Exported to the USA	13,629	12,810	6,282	

Sources: Almanac of China's Foreign Economic Relations and Trade, 1986; World Agricultural Regional Outlook, 1985, US State Department 1983.

used, and it has been estimated that the initial outlay could be recouped in three to five years. This aspect of Traditional medicine must therefore be seen as a growth point in the modernizing Chinese economy (Hillier 1983, p. 329).

Traditional Medicine in American Chinatowns[3]

A New York survey in the 1970s reviewed Chinese signs on the streets, and advertisements in six Chinese newspapers. The survey also conducted a street census uncovering twenty herbalists, five acupuncturists, and seven bone setters present in New York City's Chinatown (Chan 1976). With the tremendous population growth in Chinatowns following the 1965 rise in the quota for Oriental immigrants from 102 a year to 20,000, the number of Traditional Chinese physicians also increased (Huang 1976). Previous to 1970, the New York City Department of Health reported the presence of eighteen

Chinese healers in Chinatown. By 1973, their number had swelled to fifty. Moreover, although special herbs were difficult to obtain because of the lack of a trading agreement with the People's Republic of China before 1980, herbs could be bought in at least twenty-one herb shops, grocery stores, laundries, book stores, department stores, gift shops, and travel agencies (Chan 1976).

Utilization patterns among Chinese-Americans found, in a study of 100 Chinese American mothers, that 47 percent of them ingested one or more herbs during their pregnancy and 53 percent of them complied with at least one food taboo (Ling 1975). In addition, according to another survey, 43 percent of San Franciscan Chinese-American elderly visited a "doctor" at minimum once a month. Many of these doctors, do not have degrees since to the elderly, herbalists are also "doctors" (Carp 1976).

Other factors involved in the continuing use of Traditional medicine in the USA include: (1) limited accessibility to western care facilities; (2) a dearth of Chinese allied health personnel (nurses, medical technicians, lab technicians); (3) a poor understanding of the American health care system and the resources available; (4) language and cultural barriers; and (5) adherence to Chinese medical teachings. Further, for whatever reasons, there is evidence that some patients choose Chinese treatment for certain diseases such as rheumatism, stroke, sprains, gastrointestinal problems, anemia, fractures, and itching (Chen 1976) (Li 1972).

Such data should not be overstated because the same surveys also indicate extensive use of western medicines as well. For example, in the above survey of Chinese-American mothers, nearly 50 percent of them either did not comply with food taboos or take any herbs. In addition, in a study of 87 Chinese households in New York City's Chinatown, nearly 83 percent of them saw MDs exclusively, and only 17 percent had had some experience with Traditional healers within the past two years. No one had visited a Chinese practitioner exclusively, and no one during the preceding two years had consulted Traditional doctors more often than western physicians (Chen 1976). Moreover, although 93 percent of those surveyed stated that in the prior two years they had had some contact with Chinese pharmacology, western drugs were used in self-treatment six times out of ten, and no households took only herbs. Of course the Chen study is a limited one of only a single Chinatown, but it does indicate some continuing market for this export item from the PRC. The presence of overseas Chinese communities in many western and Asian countries certainly guarantees a continuing market for herbal medicines and Traditional remedies.

RECENT REPORTS

Recent reports from the official Chinese press continue to describe the interest in and use of Traditional medicine techniques. It is impossible to gauge from this material the extent of use. Nonetheless, it is clear that official government policy is to protect, develop and promote the use of Traditional Chinese medicine in various forms (Zhang 1985).

By 1983, China had approximately 300,000 doctors and paramedics in Traditional Chinese medicine. Between 1976 and 1983, the Ministry of Public Health conferred academic titles on 167,000 of these Traditional practitioners and promoted 1,500 of them to chief doctors in their fields. Fifty of the most famous of these doctors were elected delegates to the Sixth National People's Congress, or appointed members of the National Committee of the Chinese People's Political Consultative Conference, both significant political gestures.

In 1978, a special document was issued by the Party Central Committee reiterating the policy of developing Traditional medicine and integrating it with western medicine. Since 1978, 10,000 Traditional practitioners and herbalists have been certified through state examinations. These practitioners were already working in cooperatively owned medical settings or in their own clinics. The new constitution of 1982 includes a statement of this commitment and in that same year, the government convened a national conference of Traditional hospitals which wrote and adopted "Regulations on the Work of Hospitals of Traditional Medicine."

Official figures for 1983 stated that there were 1,000 hospitals of Traditional Chinese medicine above the county level with more than 70,000 beds, twenty-four colleges of Traditional medicine, forty-eight research institutes above the city level with more centers to be established in Shanghai, Chengden and Wuhan. Expansion of enrollments at the colleges of Traditional medicine meant that 25,000 were studying at the colleges. One hundred twenty-five Traditional specialty departments were offering post-graduate studies. The old system of apprenticeships persists as well. Advanced students can be apprenticed to "celebrated" older Traditional doctors.

This same official report states that "several thousand kinds of medicinal herbs used by Traditional doctors are attracting more and more attention from international medical organizations. This is because the vast majority of these herbs have no or little side effects. Some of them are just ordinary cereals, vegetables and fruits" (Zhang 1985, p. 20).

There continues to be scientific research carried out on the clinical efficacy of Traditional medicines either along or in combination with western medicines. These are based on clinical observation and experimental study although, as far as is known, double blind studies are not conducted. The claim remains for a "large group of effective (Traditional) medicines." These include Guan Xin No. 2 which is "90 percent effective for angina pectorals," volatile oil extracted from *Vitex negunds var cannabifolia* and *artemisia apcacea* 80 percent effective for chronic bronchitis; it is claimed that "using extracts from *Camptotheca acuminata*, wild lily and polyporus to treat cancer can prolong the lifespan of patients by five years, decrease the toxic effects of radiotherapy and chemotherapy, and enhance the body's resistance to other diseases" while extracts from *Artemisia piacea* is better than *chloroquine* for treating various types of malaria. Research on acupuncture has not only established its anesthetic properties but that it "can cure cardiovascular disease and diseases of the digestive system." By the year of 1983, nearly 300 of these scientific discoveries had received recognition through State or Ministry of Public Health national awards (Zhang 1985).

There are also examples of computerization of Traditional medicine treatments. In 1982, the Academy of Traditional Medicine began to record the diagnostic and treatment knowledge of Zhu Renkang a seventy-six year old nationally famous doctor of Chinese medicine and dermatology.

The program has been tested on 365 patient cases with a 97 percent cure rate (Zhang 1985).

Government figures for 1985 permit some insight into the growth of Traditional medicine institutions over a short time span as well as the calculation of their proportions compared to western medicine (see Table 5.3).

Overall, these figures suggest that Traditional medicine resources constitute almost 24 percent of all medical personnel now, 30 percent of the medical education institutions but, as of 1985, only 17.8 percent of medical undergraduates. This suggests that their proportion of the medical manpower pool will shrink in the future. Traditional hospital beds are 4.5 percent of total hospital beds corroborating that Traditional medicine is primarily concentrated in out-patient facilities. Traditional research institutes are approximately 8 percent of all research institutes in the country, a small enterprise but there nonetheless.

CONCLUSIONS

An unusual experiment, launched in the early years of the People's Republic of China, has saved an ancient medical tradition from extinction. That experiment has given Chinese Traditional medicine a new life, indeed a future in the modern world. However, that new life is rather more modest than may have originally been envisioned, and in a rather different form than many thought.

While herbal gardens and preparation of herbal prescriptions in the Traditional mode are found in many health facilities, evidence indicates that the more rural and less affluent facilities are more reliant on Traditional medicine than are the more urban and affluent facilities. This suggests that as the country is more able to manufacture and purchase western pharmeceuticals, the Traditional will gradually decrease in use. Visits to Traditional hospitals and medical schools also revealed that they are assimilating western techniques and technologies with considerable interest.

There is also ample evidence that Traditional recipes are being standardized and produced as patent medicines thereby changing the original character of Traditional prescribing which was highly individualized. Production is being more highly regulated than ever before. These patent medicines, along with crude drug products, are an important export item for the PRC, going mainly to Asia and Africa, but to the industrialized nations as well. Evidence of their continued but limited use can be found, for example, in American Chinatowns.

A review of recent material shows continued support for research to establish the scientific basis for Traditional medicines and techniques. While 24 percent of all medical personnel are now some sort of Traditional practitioner, only 18 percent of all medical students are in Traditional medical schools. Although there were extensive plans to educate many doctors of "integrated medicine," there are only a minute number of such senior doctors in the country today. The use of Traditional medicine seems to be concentrated primarily in ambulatory settings, although it does appear to be used pervasively for some acute abdominal conditions like appendicitis.

There will continue to be high interest in Chinese Traditional medicine for a wide variety of reasons, some clinical, some economic and some political. From a medical point of view, the curative qualities of Traditional medicine will continue to be studied and may attract further attention because of reduced side effects as well as lower costs.

To review the transformation of Chinese Traditional medicine is a rare opportunity to see the modernization process in progress. Political will, economic necessity, and cultural pride gave Traditional medicine the impetus for survival. The modernization policy is giving Chinese Traditional medicine the form of its future.

NOTES

1. The material on herbal medicines and appendicitis was prepared by Melissa Gregory, a member of the 1981 Study Group.

2. An American medical perspective on this treatment was provided by an internist at the Veterans Hospital in Ann

Arbor, Michigan (Wheatley 1981). The evacuation of the intestine, accomplished by herbs with laxative properties, was viewed by Dr Wheatley as a possibly dangerous procedure. Laxatives increase the motility of the intestine and, in the case of a ruptured appendix, the increased movement would spread infection throughout the abdominal cavity. Although this method may rid the appendix of an obstruction causing the infection, Wheatley indicated that the dangers involved outweighed the possible advantages. In principle using antibacterial agents is a good idea. However, the effectiveness of herbal bactericides that need to be absorbed through the intestinal lumen before reaching the appendix he found questionable. Increased circulation would be beneficial by increasing the number of white blood cells and immune factors reaching the appendix. Dr Wheatley noted, however, that the appendix artery is very small and during appendicitis is often already dilated and sometimes obstructed thus rendering any effects of circulation minimal.

3. The material on the use of Traditional practitioners and Traditional medicine in American Chinatowns was prepared by John Leung, a member of the 1979 study group.

TABLE 5.2
NINE HERBAL PRESCRIPTIONS FOR APPENDICITIS

PRESCRIPTION ONE

Rheum officinale	*Glycyrrhiza uralensis*
Paeonae moutan	*Lonicera japonica*
Benincasa cerifera	*Prunus persica*
Na_2SO_4	*Forsythiae suspensa*
Aralia edulis	*Aegle seporia*
Platycodon grandflorium	

Source: Acute Abdominal Condition Research Group, 1959.

PRESCRIPTION TWO

Patrinia scabiosaefolia	*Aconitum fisheri*
Pearl barley	*Lonicera japonica*
Aralia edulis	

Source: First Hospital of Kirin Province, 1959.

PRESCRIPTION THREE

Lonicera japenica   *Prunus persica*

Taraxacum officinale   *Saussurea lappa*

Patrinia scabioseafolia   *Meliae toosendan*

Forsythiae suspensa   *Paeoniae lactiflora*

Herba hedvotidis diffusa   *Rheum officinale*

Benincasa cerifera

Source: Institute for Acute Abdominal Diseases, 1977a.

PRESCRIPTION FOUR

Rheum tangaticum   *Sonchus bracyotus*

Magnolia officinalis   *Sargentodoxa cerneata*

Source: National Academy of Science, 1975.

PRESCRIPTION FIVE

Rheum tangaticum	*Paeoniae lactiflora*
Taraxacum mongolicum	*Alcebia guinata*
Lonicera Japonica	*Corydalis bulbosa*
Prunus persica	*Prunus mume*

Source: National Academy of Science, 1975.

PRESCRIPTION SIX

Lonicera japonica	*Prunus persica*
Taraxacum officinale	*Rheum officinale*
Patrinia scabiosaefolia	

Source: Institute for Acute Abdominal Diseases, 1977b.

PRESCRIPTION SEVEN

Rheum tangatieum   *Sargentodoxa cuneata*

Taraxacum mongolicum   *Magnolia officinalis*

Source: National Academy of Science, 1975.

PRESCRIPTION EIGHT

Paeoniae moutan   Na2SO4

Rheum officinale   *benincasa cerifera*

Prunus persica

Source: Hyatt, 1978.

PRESCRIPTION NINE

Zingiber officinale   *Glycyrrhiza uralensis*

Zizyphus jujuba   *Paeoniae lactiflora*

Source: Hyatt, 1978.

TABLE 5.3
Traditional Medicine Resources 1983-1985

	Total Resources (1985)	Traditional (1983)[a]	Traditional (1985)[b]	Traditional as % of all
Medical colleges and universities	116	24	24 colleges 11 faculties of higher learning	30%
Medical undergraduates	157,000	25,000	28,000	17.8%
Research Institutes (Independent and Affiliated)	680 515	48 above city level --	54 --	7.9%
Secondary Schools of Medicine and Pharmacy Students	221,000	--	--	
Total Personnel (medical doctors including western and traditional assistants)	1.413 million	1,000 above county level	336,000	23.7%
Hospitals	60,000		1,455	2.4%
Hospital Beds	2.229 million	70,000	102,000	4.5%
Senior Doctors of "Integrated Medicine"	2,036			

Sources: a Zhang, 1985.
         b PRC Embassy, 1987.

REFERENCES

Acute Abdominal Condition Research Group.
1959 Acupuncture and traditional drugs in treatment of appendicitis. Chinese Medical Journal, 79:72–76.

Almanac of China's Foreign Economic Relations and Trade
1986 Ministry of Foreign Economic Relations and Trade. China Resource Trade Consultancy, Ltd., Hong Kong, pp. 989–993.

Beijing Review
1985 Special Report: Passing on Traditional Chinese Medicine, No. 3, 21 January, p. 25.

Beijing Review
1985 "Time-Honored Pharmacy Anniversary Marked," Vol. 98, No. 3, March, p. 176.

Beijing Review
1980 "China's Ancient Pharmacy," No. 50, 15 December 1980, p. 24.

Carp, Frances M., and Eunice Kataoka.
1976 "Health Care Problems of the Elderly of San Francisco's Chinatown," The Gerontologist, Vol. 16, No. 1, Part. 1, pp. 30–38.

Chan, Chun-Wai, and Jade K. Chang.
1976 "The Role of Chinese Medicine in New York City's Chinatown," Part 1, American Journal of Chinese Medicine, Vol. 4, No. 1, pp. 31–45 and Part 2, American Journal of Chinese Medicine, Vol. 4, No. 2, pp. 129–146.

Daily Report
1982 Daily Report-China. "Pharmaceutical Figures Noted," 11 February, Vol. 1, No. 029, Annex, No. 004, K11.

Direction of Trade
1985 Direction of Trade Statistics Yearbook Annual. International Monetary Fund.

Dong-hai, Jiao.
1980 Resume of 400 cases of acute upper digestive tract bleeding treated by rhubarb alone. Pharmacology, 20 (Suppl. 1):128–130.

174

Hillier, S. M., and J. A. Jewell
  1983 Health Care and Traditional Medicine in China 1800–
    1982. Routledge and Kegan Paul, London, Boston,
    Melbourne and Henley.
Huang, Jacob Chen-Ya, and Freda Grachow.
  1976 "Health Services Dilemma: Chinatown, New York
    City," New York State Journal of Medicine, Vol. 76,
    No. 2, February, pp. 297–301.
Hyatt, Richard, and Feldman, Robert.
  1978 Chinese herbal medicine: Ancient art and modern
    medicine. New York: Schocken Books.
Institute for Acute Abdominal Diseases.
  1977a Combined Traditional Chinese and western medicine
    in acute appendicitis. Chinese Medical Journal, 3(4):266–
    269.
Institute for Acute Abdominal Diseases.
  1977b Treatment of acute appendicitis in children with
    combined Traditional and western medicine. Chinese
    Medical Journal, 3(6):373–378.
Institute for Acute Abdominal Diseases.
  1978 Treatment of acute abdominal diseases by combined
    western and Traditional medicine. Chinese Medical
    Journal, 4(1–6):11–16.
Lasagna, Louis.
  1975 Herbal pharmacology and medical therapy in the
    People's Republic of China. Annals of Internal
    Medicine. 83(6):887–893.
Li, Frederick P.
  1972 "Traditional Chinese Medicine in the United States,"
    Journal of the American Medical Association, Vol. 220,
    No. 8, 22 May, pp. 1134–1135.
Ling, Stella, Janet King, and Virginia Leung.
  1975 "Diet, Growth, and Cultural Food Habits in Chinese-
    American Infants," American Journal of Chinese
    Medicine, Vol. 3, No. 2, pp. 125–132.
National Academy of Sciences.
  1975 Herbal pharmacology in the People's Republic of China:
    A trip report of the American herbal pharmacology
    delegation. Washington, DC.

175

People's Republic of China Embassy
1987 "A Brief Introduction on China's Medical and Health
Services." Document provided by the Embassy of the
People's Republic of China, Washington, D.C. Received
February 1987, undated, pp. 12–19.
Shibata S.
1979 The Chemistry of Chinese Drugs, American Journal of
Chinese Medicine, Summer, 7(2):103–41.
Study Journals
1979 and 1981 Study Journals of the University of Michigan-
Dearborn/Michigan State University Health Care Study
Groups. August 1979 and July 1981. Complete
transcriptions of all information gathered, all questions
asked and all answers provided. Available from the
author upon request.
US State Department
1983 China: Background Notes. Bureau of Public Affairs,
December.
Wheatley, Charles, MD.
1981 An interview was held with Dr. Wheatley, an internist
at the Veterans Administration Hospital, Ann Arbor,
Michigan. September.
World Agriculture
1985 World Agriculture Regional Outlook: Eastern Europe,
China, Subsharan Africa, ASI:85.
Zhang Gongyuan
1985 "Passing on Traditional Chinese Medicine," Beijing
Review, No. 1–25, January – June, pp. 20–26.

6
MODERNIZATION AND HEALTH CARE IN THE PEOPLE'S REPUBLIC OF CHINA: AN OVERVIEW

It was striking innovations like Barefoot Doctors and the use of Traditional medicine that brought the health care system of the People's Republic of China (PRC) to worldwide attention. As creative as these policies were and are, they only tell part of the story about health care delivery in the PRC. Time, and cooler, more informed research and descriptions have become available. They tell a more complex, more subtle and equally fascinating story about developments in the Chinese health care system, particularly its condition and fate during the current period of "modernization" in that country.[1]

China was a devastated country when the Communists took over the government in 1948, poverty-striken, rife with disease and with severely limited medical resources. However, health policy issues that China's leaders have had to face are basically no different than those faced in other countries be they western developed nations or agricultural and industrializing Third World nations. These are issues that have to do with equity, access to care, distribution of care, cost containment and quality of care. Each nation works on these issues in the context of its own unique historical culture, political system and economic conditions. And it generally

A version of this article appeared in The Journal of Medical Practice Management, Winter 1987, Vol. 2, No. 3 and is reprinted with permission. The figure renderings in Ch. 6 are used through the courtesy of Waverly Press, Baltimore, Maryland.

works on them in an evolutionary fashion. This latter is where the People's Republic of China goes its unique way. At seminal points in its modern history, health policy and revolutionary ideology embraced in a remarkable burst of energy to try to accelerate change. This happened twice: in the immediate revolutionary fervor arising out of the success of the communist revolution in 1949 which set the original direction for health policy, and in the Great Proletarian Cultural Revolution (1965 – 1968) and its immediate aftermath. It was during the early period that the first attempts to integrate Traditional and modern medicine took place. It was during the Cultural Revolution that the Barefoot Doctor program was launched.

The Chinese health care system is more, however, than these two features and what is of particular interest is what is happening to the system – including Traditional medicine and Barefoot Doctors – today, during this period of modernization in the People's Republic of China when pragmatism rather than ideological fervor dominates the governance of the country.

China, containing one billion people (and a quarter of the world's population) organizes its health care system with relationships to important political units. These encompass its twenty-one provinces and three centrally governed large cities, counties within the provinces and communes (now villages). Each has various health related responsibilities that reflect general health policy which is formulated by the National Ministry of Health in Beijing. It is a relatively decentralized system with financing and delivery left to local political units on the county and village levels. Figures 6.1 and 6.2 provide a picture of the urban and rural organizational structure of the system.

Experts estimate that the PRC spends between 2 to 3 percent of GNP on its health care system, a percentage some-what higher than its Asian neighbors (World Bank 1984). From a financing point of view, the PRC does not have a unified insurance system but rather three separate insurance funds (which cover targeted populations), see Figure 6.3. About two percent of the population is covered by a "public medical insurance"; this includes government workers and political cadre, but not their families. A second plan covers an additional 10 to 12 percent of workers in government-owned factories and farms. The rural population is covered by the "co-operative medical service" set up on a local basis but subject to the exigencies of crop failures and success. About 48 percent of the communes or villages are thought to have the service in place. The decentralized nature of funding and of administration means that services and facilities are uneven around the country. The problems of distribution of services and personnel have been chronic and constitute the single most difficult challenge to Chinese health policy to this day. All policy innovations and programs attempt to diminish the inequalities in the health system.

Nonetheless, by any standards, the strides in health and health services improvements since 1949 are extraordinary. And when the PRC is compared today to other Asian countries, its accomplishments are impressive.

Historical Background

The evolution of the PRC health care system is rooted in historical events and cultural traditions as well as Maoist ideology and the current priorities of modernization. Nineteenth century missionary doctors introduced western medical practices which often addressed medical problems with which Traditional medicine was unable to cope. The foundations of the county hospital system were laid during the twentieth century Republic and Nationalist periods which also established model village centers. The experiences of the Red Army during the extended civil war in the 1930s and 1940s suggested the possibility of giving primitive medical training to peasants and peasant soldiers. The Red Army also recognized the uses of Traditional doctors, Traditional medical techniques and herbs where nothing else was available and saw the dependence and belief of the peasants in these resources. The leaders of the Red Army also recognized the power of revolutionary fervor in overcoming formidable odds.

During the fifteen-year period after the revolution, what is known among China scholars as the "socialist transformation," this fervor and these experiences were used to launch mass health campaigns that were successful in eliminating venereal disease, controlling pests, reducing the incidence of schistosomiasis and subduing a wide variety of infectious disease. There were many efforts to integrate Traditional and western medicine during this period. When the Cultural Revolution was launched in 1965, as Mao tried to regain political power and rekindle revolutionary zeal, the Barefoot Doctor program was launched and renewed emphasis on health care delivery in the rural areas stressed. Since the early 1980s, the new commitment to modernization has meant additional priorities for health care delivery: an interest in advanced medical technology and professionalization, what has been called the Great Leap Westward.

How has the modernization period affected the health care system, particularly the innovations that marked the earlier developments after the Revolution?

The Fate of Traditional Medicine

The western world was intrigued with Mao's attempt to preserve Chinese Traditional medicine (Chung-i) and bring it into the modern world. Some romanticized this health policy of the People's Republic of China and saw it as an effort to retain an ancient and venerable traditional treasure that offered superior approaches to medical care. Others regarded it as a form of foolish madness, preserving an unscientific and useless form of feudal medical practice. A closer study of Mao's motivations in promoting the integration of Traditional and western medicine revealed a complex of pragmatic motivations.

These included a desperate need for medical personnel, lack of western pharmaceutical resources and little capital to purchase them, a recognition that the vast rural population believed in Traditional medicine, and a desire to help rebuild national pride by promoting this aspect of traditional culture. What Mao hoped to accomplish was the modernization of Traditional medicine itself. As early as 1944, well before the success of the Revolution, he stated, "To surrender to the old style is wrong; to abolish or discard is wrong; our responsibility is to unite those of the old style that can be used, and to help stimulate and reform them."

Observational research conducted by visitors to the PRC during the 1970s and 1980s indicated that the use of

Traditional medicines and techniques was highly selective (see Chapter Two in this book). While acupuncture clinics are found in all the western-style medical facilities and used for various chronic conditions and a limited number of herbal prescriptions used for certain acute illnesses, this is all carried out under the supervision of western-style doctors. In the Traditional hospitals and medical schools, western-style doctors are also in charge and the approaches include extensive use of modern medicines and diagnostic techniques and western-style medical theory. Applicants to the twenty-four Traditional medical colleges have to pass the same national examination required of all medical school applicants. This emphasizes chemistry, math, physics and a foreign language.

There is considerable evidence that Traditional practitioners and approaches are the most extensively used in more remote areas of the country. The distant rural countryside hospitals have major in- and out-patient Traditional departments and rely on Traditional approaches more than in the urban areas. For example, many rural county hospitals and commune district hospitals have extensive herbal gardens, growing 180 to 300 different herbs. These medicinal gardens are tended by elderly Traditional doctors or herbalists. Such locations also have facilities for drying and storing herbs and making their own pills and other medications. Economic necessity remains a powerful stimulant for such practices.

A visit, in 1981, to Shanghai's Traditional Medicine Factory #1 provided insight into how herbal medicines are being transformed today. This factory had originally been organized by bringing together six old herbal workshops. The current director of the factory was originally the head of one of these workshops and got his training as a child apprentice to an elderly Traditional herbalist. Today his staff includes herbalists with similar backgrounds as well as modern engineers and pharmacists (see Chapter Five in this book for details).

This factory has pooled its Traditional recipes and now manufactures 230 of them as standardized, over-the-counter medicine. It has chosen those recipes that have been the most popular and efficacious. Modern factory assembly line manufacturing techniques are utilized with random sample quality control. Its products are sold throughout China and

Asia. It is also possible to find medicines from Shanghai Factory #1 in the Chinatowns of the United States and Canada.

What it sells is no longer Traditional medicine in the strict sense. A Traditional doctor would change recipes or prescriptions every few days during the course of an illness to reflect changes in the patient's condition. The medicines produced at Shanghai Traditional Medicine Factory #1 eliminate this approach and 'freeze' the recipes into a single form. What is happening to herbal medicine at the factory is its transformation into patent medicine. Overall, China produces more than 3,000 kinds of patent Traditional medicines and they are an important export item for the country.

The Academy of Traditional Medicine in Beijing, established in the 1970s, is the major research institution in the country, supplying modern scientific methods to Traditional medicine. It systematically studies its clinical practice, the pharmacological efficacy of herbs, and the mechanisms of moxibustion and acupuncture. Acupuncture continues to be used as a treatment modality for some 300 different diseases including acute viral hepatitis, bacterial dysentery, bronchial asthma and especially for pain.

The effort to preserve Chinese Traditional medicine and combine it with modern medicine in the PRC was the idea of a radical, powerful and pragmatic political leader. This health policy decision was based on economic necessity, political realism and the desire to impose scientific modernism on a traditional element of Chinese culture. It produced a unique health care innovation and provides a model for other agricultural, Third World nations.

Thirty-five years later, this policy has proved fruitful. The significant numbers of Traditional doctors in the early 1950s provided an important resource of practitioners that continues to be developed. Economically, it has provided medicinal and treatment resources for the rural areas of China which had, and continue to have, little money to purchase modern pharmaceuticals and equipment. It has also provided an income to the nation as an important foreign trade item.

From a political point of view, Traditional practitioners have provided a link to the peasants in the modernization process. As the Traditional practitioners have absorbed modern medical knowledge, they have passed it on in services to their patients. In this way, they are a bridge between a tradition that was trusted by the peasant and a new, modernized China that the current leadership of the country is struggling to build.

Finally, the application of modern research to Chung-i has permitted a more accurate understanding of what is useful and efficacious in Traditional medicine by modern scientific standards. With his integration policy, Mao really wanted to bring Chung-i into the modern world; his goal is on its way to being accomplished.

Barefoot Doctors and the Professionalization Process

China's Barefoot Doctor (BFD) program is undergoing significant change. In 1977, the number of BFDs began to decline. First from 1,760,000 to 1,575,000 with 185,000 dismissed as incompetent or leaving for other reasons. Now it has been estimated that 40 percent of the pool of BFDs are no longer practicing. Standards for training are rising with increased emphasis on medical work and a two-level system of examinations has been instituted. This includes a BFD competency test and a more advanced examination to receive certification as a "country or village doctor" for the best students. A small percentage of medical school places are reserved for the most promising Barefoot Doctors. Overall, current policy indicates Barefoot Doctors are to become the equivalent of three-year medical school graduates (assistant doctors), be full-time practitioners and receive salaries instead of workpoints (see Chapter One).

In June of 1965, on the eve of the Great Proletariate Cultural Revolution, Chairman Mao announced a new health policy: a Barefoot Doctor program designed to deal with the continuing shortage of physicians for China's vast rural population. Mao mandated that hundreds of thousands of rural peasants, chosen by their work comrades, would be given several months of rudimentary medical training. They would continue in agricultural labor part-time in addition to serving the elementary health care needs of their fellow workers.

This was a remarkable idea in its daring and in its risks. Based on early efforts during the 1930s Rural Reconstruction Movement and small 1950s experiments near Shanghai, the Barefoot Doctor policy appeared to have a number of purposes: (1) It created a new health provider category to deal with both the continuing shortage and maldistribution of physicians. Despite successful efforts both to increase the number of medical students and to disperse them to rural areas, the stark doctor shortage so evident in 1949 at the point of liberation continued, as did the urban clustering of the medical profession. (2) Mao's anger with the medical profession, one of the urban elites he had always mistrusted, had reached new heights. He attacked the Ministry of Health with intense fury in 1965. It was one of the power bases of his political enemies and represented resistance to his conception of the principles of continuing revolution. By creating a large cadre of health workers from outside the world of professional medical knowledge, he moved to undercut professional control of medical work.

Third, Mao and the CCP still had unfulfilled, and important, obligations to the rural masses who had made the revolution a success. The Barefoot Doctor concept was a bold move to make good on promises in a dramatic, egalitarian manner: taking young peasants, training them, yet leaving them to continue working alongside of their comrades in the fields. This ingenious idea would cause a minimum drain on agricultural workers where all hands are needed. It also fortified the concept of equal status between practitioner and patient. (4) Further, the policy emphasized local autonomy and initiatives, consistent with the 1960s thrust for decentralization. (5) Finally, it was a concrete example of the Cultural Revolution's emphasis on practical work rather than theoretical education.

This medical manpower policy also reflected a personification of Mao's original principles of health work. Barefoot Doctors were to be trained in both western and Traditional medical knowledge, to practice preventive medicine, to organize their fellows in mass health campaigns and serve the health needs of people at the grass roots level.

After its implementation, the major concerns about the BFD program were tri-fold; the quality of care the Barefoot Doctors could offer, the unevenness of education they received and the diverse demands put on them. Observational research revealed that the Barefoot Doctors with the least training often had the greatest demands to provide services. This happened particularly in the remote rural areas which needed their services the most because of their distance from the more developed services of the cities. The upgrading efforts are a current attempt to address this problem.

The unevenness in both quality and quantity of Barefoot Doctors around the country will no doubt slow the professionalization process. As has been pointed out and substantiated, variability will continue to be related to economic and geographic factors unless there is long-term central government subsidy to the program. Barefoot Doctors continue to be vulnerable to the exigencies of agricultural output and local conditions. A further complication are the incentives for private plots in the rural areas and this helps to account for the large decline in numbers of BFDs by 40 percent. It may be more profitable to work these plots than practice as a village doctor.

Mao's boldness in 1965 created a new pool of medical workers in an effort to deal with the continuing physician distribution problems in the PRC. The current government is building on the 1960s effort by upgrading the Barefoot Doctors, moving them towards professionalization. Like the Traditional practitioners, they will slowly move towards a western model in another innovative use of available resources.

Development of the Rural Health Care System

Both the Barefoot Doctor program and the Traditional medicine policy are closely tied to the development of China's rural health care system. This has been a major priority since the early 1950s and remains a continuing challenge today in the struggle to improve delivery and increase resources in the many poor rural areas of the country. Although emphasis on rural care was clear at the First National Health Congress, held in 1950, a variety of problems has frustrated the full evolution of the rural system (see Chapter Three). This included the belief that existing resources in the urban areas should be strengthened first, the lack of central government

funds to assist the weakest areas, and decentralized financing
and authority. Figure 6.4 presents the urban-rural differences
in health expenditures.

With the drive to collectivize the countryside during the
mid-1950s "Great Leap Forward," promises of a rural network
of health care delivery became most pressing. The existence of
local medical units would make the commune system more
attractive to the rural citizenry and be tangible evidence of the
Chinese Communist Party's commitment to their well-being.
Progress was slow and reports of the inadequacy of rural health
care resources persisted into the 1960s.

The Great Leap Forward paradoxically forced the rural
health care system into a real dilemma. With the Great Leap
Forward came an elimination of all fees at the time of treatment. Predictably, health care costs skyrocketed upward and
imposed even greater problems upon the already financially
strapped rural system. Increasing costs, along with other
political and economic problems, lead to a decrease in brigade
cooperative health funds. The result was a cutback in available
services with the eventual erosion of free (collectively-run)
commune clinics during this period. The inadequate care being
delivered to China's rural peasants laid the groundwork for
Mao's 1965 effort to redirect emphasis to rural health needs.
Not only did he create the BFD program but he also pushed
the program to send urban physicians out to the rural
countryside to practice and teach health care. This period sees
an acceleration of the organization of delivery units at all levels
of the rural political and economic structure.

Out in the Countryside

The rural health and medical system as observed in the
early 1980s is basically a county five-tier system. The first
tier, staffed primarily by the Barefoot Doctor and assisted by
midwives and health aides, is the production brigade health
station. It is at this level where the peasant often first comes
into contact with the medical system. If the patient's problem
is beyond the scope of the station, the patient is ideally referred
up to the next level of the system, the commune hospital.
Staffed with western-style and Traditional doctors, nurses and

other health workers and sometimes with a limited number of in-patient beds, the commune hospital is equipped to handle somewhat more difficult cases. The third level of the system is a more sophisticated commune hospital known as the District (or Central) Commune Hospital which serves its own commune and four to six others by offering specialized services. The fourth tier is the County Hospital which is the most elaborate of the strictly rural facilities. The County Bureaus of Public Health are emerging as a fifth tier in the system, clearly functioning on the health rather than medical side of the system but with increasing responsibility for managing the entire county health care system.

What these county systems look like, however, varies greatly around the country. Among the counties visited by this author in 1979 and 1981 was one in an area (Nong An) never before observed by foreigners where there was a significant emphasis on Traditional approaches and heavy demands made on relatively limited facilities. In significant contrast was a wealthy rural county, Ye Hsien, with an almost exclusively western-style orientation, well developed and expanding facilities, excellent state financial support yet providing essentially the same level of care as Nong An. The commune health facilities in other geographically diverse areas, both rural and suburban that were visited also reflected a wide diversity of ability to provide adequate care. The poorer the commune, the more limited the health and medical facilities and the greater the reliance on Traditional approaches.

Furthermore, a comprehensive study of hospital care (Henderson and Cohen 1982) by two American researchers who worked in a Chinese hospital for six months found that rural patients had serious problems of access to tertiary care compared to urban patients.

Reports on the impact of other modernization agricultural policies like emphasizing family endeavors over collective endeavors have created new problems. Hsiao (1984) reports that about 80 percent of brigades are now engaged in the household production system and that this has caused the collective welfare and health system to suffer. The decline of the cooperative medical system has meant that the peasants must bear the financial burden of illness. He states:

In the health area, the central government finances only the national hospitals, research institutes and medical schools which report directly to the central government. Each province or county is responsible for its own public services, including health care, education, and welfare. Thus, a prosperous county may be able to provide generous health-care facilities, and a poor county may have to settle for less. Such differences accentuate the already uneven distribution of health services in the rural areas (Hsiao NEJM:933).

Western-Style Medicine

Despite the emphasis on Traditional or semi-Traditional medicine in the rural areas, western-style medicine is, of course, the major mode of medical practice in mainland China and dominates the health service in the urban areas of the country (Beijing Review 1980–1985; Chinese Medical Journal 1980–1985). Visitors to urban hospitals and clinics note immediately, however, that the technology is dated, some of it identifiable as circa 1920s and 1930s. Although the medical specialists have kept up with changes in procedures through the scientific literature, their ability to implement new methods has been greatly hampered by a lack of the most contemporary equipment. This is beginning to change in the most advanced medical centers in Beijing and Shanghai, for example, as advanced technologies are imported and adapted. Further, hundreds of senior medical scientists and graduate students have been going abroad to study medicine and related fields to bring advanced diagnostic and treatment techniques back to China.

China currently has 116 "advanced medical schools" (Cheng 1984). The overwhelming majority are based on a five-year curriculum that includes medicine, public health, dentistry, and pediatrics, with 10 to 20 percent of the study devoted to Traditional medicine. Also, a few of the schools offer an eight-year program for the most advanced specialists. Six of the 116 advanced medical schools are designated key medical colleges, receive priority in resources, and the best medical graduates. All the medical schools, which were highly limited during the Cultural Revolution, are moving towards higher standards and more resources. This includes those which emphasize Traditional medicine but whose curriculum is at least 30 percent based on western-style medicine. There are an additional 550 secondary medical schools for the allied health occupations.

A quotation from a 1980 interview with Qian Xinzhong, Minister of Health, sums up well the state of western-style medicine and medical education:

> By modern standards, medical science in our country is still not highly developed. Its equipment is outdated and its development in various regions, in towns and in the countryside is very uneven . . . our goal is to elevate medical science and technology in our country to the world's advanced levels, to provide our hospitals and clinics in both urban and rural areas with modern technology and equipment and run them in a scientific way; also we must build up a high professional contingent with a good grasp of modern medical science and technology . . . (Qian 1980:17).

Other Manifestations of the Modernization Efforts

By the end of 1984, the Chinese Academy of Sciences had sent 3,200 scholars, over half with health and medical interests, abroad for advanced study (Summaries 1980–1985). There is high interest in bringing back to China the latest treatment and diagnostic techniques. Those who return are considered to be in the vanguard of their fields and take on leading clinical and research positions. China has also imported a small amount of advanced medical technology like CT scanners which are placed in selected tertiary care centers. It is producing its own medical equipment and supplies as well, but in limited areas.

The move toward advanced medical technology will not be fast nor will it be easy. As the author of a study of a critical care unit at a Chinese urban hospital stated, there is a continuing tension over scarce resources.

... what kind of balance should ideally be struck between supporting the predominantly rural public health programs ... and fostering development of greater competence to apply the knowledge and skills of modern medicine to the treatment of patients in medical institutions staffed by highly trained professionals that will probably have to be located largely in cities? (Fox 1982:704–705).

It is particularly interesting to note that the Minister of Health, since 1981, officially began to encourage private enterprise in medicine (Xin 1985). Retired doctors are now permitted to set up fee-for-service private practices in their homes, in clinics or drug stores. Private house calls have been authorized. The hope is that these will help reduce utilization pressure on government facilities.

In the same spirit, the Ministry authorized collectives and individuals to run medical businesses "for profit." These could be drug stores or clinics. There is also now the possibility that state-owned clinics and hospitals could be "contracted out" for management. According to Xin (1985), 80,000 private doctors were practicing in China and have set up maternity wards, first aid stations and small private hospitals. There is active encouragement for local communities to start new hospitals and medical schools.

The 1985 report states,

The increase in private practice is much lower in the cities than in the rural areas. However, the limited number of private doctors is already playing an important role in diverting patients from the overtaxed public hospitals in Beijing and Wuhan. There has been a push for more home care, particularly for the chronically ill. The large cities and five or six provinces are reported to be promoting 'home beds' and a variety of home services.

There are signs of increased research and programs in occupation health and workplace hazards. While visits to a small number of factories in 1979 and 1981 revealed very little in the way of safety programs, there has been a national effort since the early 1980s to encourage factories to introduce preventive measures. A national research and education center or "labor hygiene" and occupational disease has now been established.

A *Beijing Review* interview, in 1984, with the Ministry of Health reflects current policy priorities and they reiterate the policies set in the early 1980s at the beginning of the modernization period. These include an emphasis on local hospital development, house calls, private practice, continued support of rural hospitals by urban units and the upgrading of Barefoot Doctors. Improved training of all medical personnel and upgrading medical schools was stressed. "Prevention First" and maternal and child care improvements remain major commitments. The list itself indicates what areas are felt still to be deficient.

Overall, the evidence suggests that the major innovations of the revolutionary periods—integration of Traditional and western medicine, the Barefoot Doctor program, the emphasis on rural development—are continuing as priorities in the current period of modernization. But modernization has now brought professionalization for the BFD, more rigorous standards of science applied to Traditional medicine and its standardization. Problems of rural inequities continue and the rural medical co-operatives may be faltering. Now, official policy suggests an effort to build a system of private care alongside the public one as part of the general emphasis on private initiatives. The revolutionary innovations have not been repudiated but they are clearly being transformed.

The problem of equity haunts the Chinese health care system just as it haunts western systems. Tremendous strides were taken to improve care and public health. The statistics on birth and mortality rates, facilities and personnel comparing 1950 to 1980, speak for themselves (Tables 6.1 to 6.3). But the problems remain enormous and will continue, as the system now emphasizes improving quality of care.

The Chinese health care system has emerged as a powerful model for other Third World nations. Against terrible odds, an innovative approach to care has emerged, driven by political ideology and determination, making creative use of available resources, now continuing its development under a more pragmatic philosophy. The balance of revolutionary zeal and modernization pragmatism reflects the pattern of dichotomies found in many aspects of Chinese culture and history. The health care system owes much to both dynamics, and pays a price for each.

NOTES

1. A certain portion of the material in this chapter is based on general scrutiny of *Beijing Review*, *The Chinese Medical Journal and Summaries of Mainland China Press* between 1980 and 1985 and is referenced in this fashion, a style utilized in the version of this article that appeared in the *Journal of Medical Practice Management*. Readers desiring specific citations should contact the author.

TABLE 6.1
The PRC National Birth and Mortality Rates

	Pre-liberation	1949	1952	1957	1965	1978	1982
Birth rate (unit/1,000)	35.0	36.0	37.0	34.0	37.9	18.3	21.1
Mortality rate (unit/1,000)	25.0	20.0	17.0	10.8	9.5	6.3	6.6

Source: Beijing Review 1983, No. 46, 14 November, 23-26.

TABLE 6.2
Hospital Beds and Technical Workers Per 1,000 People Throughout the PRC

	1949	1957	1965	1975	1980	1982
Hospital beds	0.15	0.46	1.06	1.74	2.02	2.03
City	0.63	2.08	3.78	4.61	4.70	4.76
Countryside	0.05	0.14	0.51	1.23	1.48	1.46
Technical medical workers	0.93	1.61	2.11	2.24	2.85	3.11
City	1.87	3.60	5.37	6.92	8.03	8.63
Countryside	0.73	1.22	1.46	1.41	1.81	1.95
Doctors and practitioners of Traditional Chinese and Western medicine	0.67	0.84	1.05	0.95	1.17	1.29
City	0.70	1.30	2.22	2.66	3.22	3.59
Countryside	0.66	0.76	0.82	0.65	0.76	0.81
Doctors of Traditional Chinese and Western medicine	0.58	0.64	0.70	0.57	0.72	0.85
City	0.54	0.86	1.41	1.61	2.14	2.53
Countryside	0.59	0.59	0.56	0.38	0.44	0.50
Senior nurses and nurses	0.06	0.20	0.32	0.41	0.47	0.56
City	0.25	0.94	1.45	1.74	1.83	2.03
Countryside	0.02	0.05	0.10	0.18	0.20	0.25

Source: Beijing Review 1983, No. 46, 14 November, pp. 23-26.

195

TABLE 6.3
Number of Professional Medical Workers in the PRC

	1949	1957	1965	1975	1980	1982
Total	541,240	1,254,372	1,872,335	2,593,517	3,534,707	3,957,804
Technical workers	505,040	1,039,203	1,531,595	2,057,068	2,798,241	3,142,943
Doctors of Traditional Chinese medicine (including those with secondary medical school education)	276,000	337,022	321,430	228,635	262,185	302,791
Pharmacists of Traditional Chinese medicine		53,505	71,848	86,201	106,963	149,231
Senior technical workers (doctors and pharmacists of western medicine and senior nurses	38,875	78,875	203,402	318,488	502,022	699,380
Middle-rank technical workers (practitioners and pharmacists of western medicine with secondary medical school education, nurses and midwives)	103,277	341,637	619,870	938,353	1,174,435	1,223,238
Junior technical workers	86,888	228,169	315,045	485,391	752,636	777,303
No. of doctors and practitioners of both Traditional Chinese and western medicine	363,400	546,296	762,804	877,716	1,153,234	1,307,205

Source: Beijing Review, 1983, No. 46, 14 November, pp. 23-26.

Figure 6.1
URBAN Health Care System

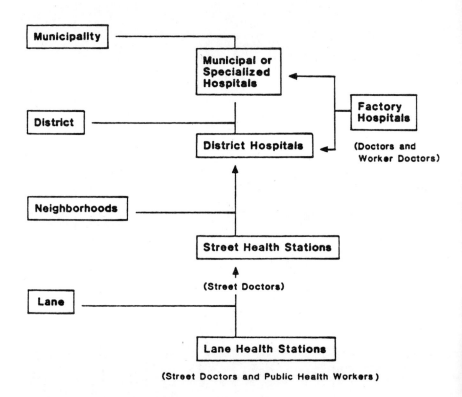

Source: Teh-wei Hu, 1984.

Figure 6.2
RURAL Health Care System

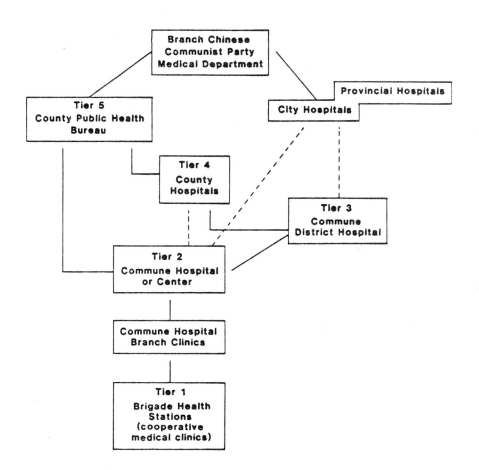

Figure 6.3
Distribution of Chinese Population by Insurance Status,
1981

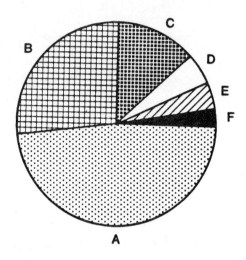

INSURANCE STATUS

A	Rural Cooperative Insurance	48%
B	Uninsured	29%
C	Labor Insurance	12%
D	Collective Industry Insurance	5%
E	Commune Industry Insurance	4%
F	Government Insurance	2%

Source: The World Bank, 1984, p. 65.

Figure 6.4
Urban-Rural Differentials in Recurrent Health Expenditures, 1981

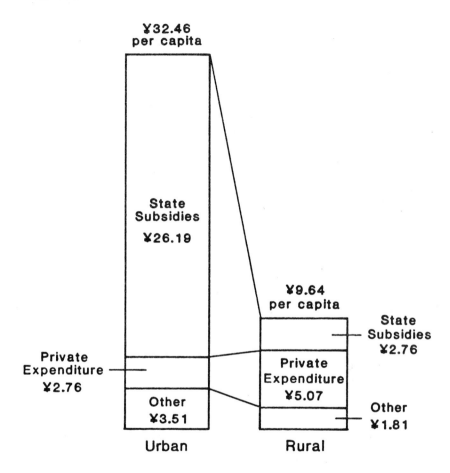

Source: The World Bank, 1984, p. 65.

200

REFERENCES

Beijing Review
  1980–1985.
Cheng Z-f.
  1984 Evolution of medical education in China. Chinese
    Medical Journal, 97:435–442.
Chinese Medical Journal
  1980–1985.
Fox, Reneé C., and Swazey, Judith P.
  1982 "Critical Care at Tianjin's First Central Hospital and
    the Fourth Modernization," Science, Vol. 217, 20 August,
    pp. 700–705.
Henderson, Gail, and Myron S. Cohen, MD.
  1982 "Health Care in the People's Republic of China: A
    View from Inside the System," American Journal of Public
    Health, November, Vol. 72, No. 11, pp. 1238–1244.
Hsiao, William C.
  1984 Special Report: Transformation of Health Care in
    China, New England Journal of Medicine, 5 April,
    pp. 932–936.
Hu, Teh-wei.
  1984 Health services in the People's Republic of China. In
    Comparative Health Systems, Marshall Raffel, (Ed.), Penn
    State University Press.
Qian, Xinzhong
  1980 Interview, "Medical and Health Service," by Lin Yang.
    Beijing Review, No. 25, 23 June, pp. 17–20.
"Summaries of Mainland China Press"
  1980–1985.
The World Bank.
  1984 China: The Health Sector, A World Bank Country
    Study, Washington, DC.
Xin
  1985 "Boosting Medical and Health Projects," Beijing
    Review, No. 23, 10 June, pp. 4–5.

APPENDIX :
LOCATIONS AND INSTITUTIONS VISITED
BY STUDY GROUPS, 1979 AND 1981

TRADITIONAL HOSPITALS

Shenyang College of Traditional Medicine and Hospital—1979

Shanghai Lung Hua Traditional Hospital—1981

PHARMACEUTICAL FACTORY

Shanghai 1st Chinese Medical Works—1981

Shenyang Northeast Pharmaceutical Factory—1979

PHARMACIES

Harbin—street pharmacy—1979

TsingTao—Chinese Drug Collecting Station—1981

TsingTao—street pharmacy—1981

SANITORIA

TsingTao Workers Sanitorium—1981

Harbin Workers Convalescent Home—1979

NEIGHBORHOODS

TsingTao #2 Yenan Road Neighborhood Health Clinic—1981

Shanghai Si Ping Workers Residential Area Health Clinic—1981

Beijing—Moon Temple Gate Neighborhood Lane Station—1979

COMMUNE HOSPITALS

5th May—Suburban Shenyang—1979

Ye County Commune—rural—1981

MaLu Commune—Suburban Shanghai—1981

Shin Hua Commune—Suburban Canton—1981

KaiAn (District Commune Hospital)—rural—1979

COUNTY HOSPITALS

Nong An—1979

Ye County—1981

PRODUCTION BRIGADES

Chei-Liang Brigade—Ye County—1981

Dong Fang Hong Production Brigade—Jinan—1981

PUBLIC HEALTH BUREAUS

Harbin—urban—1979

Ye County—rural—1981

MEDICAL SCHOOLS AND TEACHING HOSPITALS

China Medical University and Teaching Hospital—Shenyang—1979

Harbin Medical University and Teaching Hospital—#2—Harbin—1979

FACTORY HOSPITALS

Beijing—Mandarin Construction and Tool Plant Clinic— 1979

Shenyang—NE Pharmaceutical Factory Hospital—1979

Harbin—Film Projector Factory—doctors—1979

Chang Chun—Number 1 Motor Vehicle Plant Clinic—1979

TsingTao—Locomotive Factory Hospital—1981

Wai Fong—Cotton Factory Hospital—1981

CITY HOSPITAL

Tong Rein—Beijing—1979

CHINA MEDICAL ASSOCIATION—1979

HOME FOR THE ELDERLY—FUSHEN—1979

SHANGHAI SCHISTOSOMIASIS COMMITTEE—1981

INDEX

abortificients, 138
abortion, 92, 126–128, 130, 135
Academia Sinica, 137
Academy of Traditional Medicine, 157–158, 164–165, 182
acupressure, 57
acupressure tooth extraction, 58
acupuncture, 13, 18–19, 36–37, 43, 47–48, 52, 54, 57–59, 61–64, 66–67, 84–85, 149–150, 156, 161–162, 164, 180–182
acupuncturist, 78–79
acute abdomines, 36, 49, 54, 61, 72
administrative villages, 134–135
advanced-care hospital, 12
Affiliated clinic, 79
agricultural worker, 9–10, 184
agriculture, 125
All China Association of Traditional Chinese Medicine, 48
American health care system, 8, 72
American Medical Association, 154
anatomy, 14–15, 57, 64
anemia, 137–138, 162
anesthesia, 92
anesthesia, acupuncture, 57–58, 63, 66, 85, 149–150, 164
angina pectoral, 164
anthraquinones, 155
antibiotics, 156
aplastic anemia, 55–56
appendicitis, 10–11, 36, 51–52, 54, 59, 84–86, 92, 149–152, 154–155
Artemisia apiacea, 164
arterial disease, 151–152
arthritis, 47, 83, 152
arthritis, rheumatic, 151–152
assert party control, 39
'Assimilation', 44–45
assimilative, 61
assistant doctor, 5, 7–8, 11, 14, 20, 99
asthma, 182